Other monographs in the series,
Major Problems in Pathology:

Published

Evans and Cruickshank: *Epithelial Tumours of the Salivary Glands*

Mottet: *Histopathologic Spectrum of Regional Enteritis and Ulcerative Colitis*

Whitehead: *Mucosal Biopsy of the Gastrointestinal Tract*

Forthcoming

Beckwith and D'Angio: *Renal Tumors in Infants and Children*

Hadfield: *Pathology of Brain Tumors*

Hartsock: *Diagnostic Histopathology of Lymph Nodes*

Kempson: *Uterine Tumors*

Lee and Ellis: *Bone Marrow Biopsy Pathology*

Mackay: *Soft Tissue Tumors*

Melnick: *Histochemistry Applied to Pathology*

Sagebiel: *Histopathologic Diagnosis of Melanotic Lesions of Skin*

Striker, Cutler and Quadracci: *Use and Interpretation of Renal Biopsy*

Thompson: *Oesophageal Lesions*

Thurlbeck: *Chronic Obstructive Lung Disease*

J. TREVOR HUGHES, M.A., D. Phil. (Oxford), M.D. (Manchester), F.R.C.P. (Edinburgh), M.R.C.Path.

Consultant Neuropathologist, United Oxford Hospitals;
Clinical Lecturer in Neuropathology, University of Oxford

PATHOLOGY
OF
MUSCLE

Volume IV in the Series
MAJOR PROBLEMS IN PATHOLOGY

James L. Bennington, M.D., *Consulting Editor*

Chairman, Department of Pathology
Children's Hospital of San Francisco
San Francisco, California

W. B. Saunders Company, Philadelphia, London, Toronto,

W. B. Saunders Company: West Washington Square
Philadelphia, Pa. 19105

12 Dyott Street
London, WC1A   1DB

833 Oxford Street
Toronto, Ontario M8Z 5T9, Canada

Pathology of Muscle   ISBN 0-7216-4827-4

Print No.:   9   8   7   6   5   4   3   2

EDITOR'S FOREWORD

Use of the muscle biopsy for the evaluation of neuromuscular disease dates back over one hundred years. In spite of extensive experience with this technique, the greatest progress in our ability to interpret and diagnose even the most commonly encountered diseases of muscle has come during the last decade—largely through the application of new technologies to the study of muscle. Histochemical analysis and electron microscopy have helped to demonstrate enzymatic defects and structural changes not recognizable by routine methods of histologic processing and staining. Thus, new diseases and syndromes have been discovered and what were thought to be well-established entities redefined.

Dr. Hughes has contributed greatly to our understanding of muscle pathology through his research and many publications in this field. This comprehensive and timely monograph, drawn from his vast experience, concisely reviews the clinical findings and morphologic changes seen in the various diseases of muscle.

The proper evaluation of the muscle biopsy requires a team effort of clinician, surgeon and pathologist. Each member of this team, whether it be the pediatrician, neurologist, surgeon, pathologist, geneticist or histochemist, will find *Pathology of Muscle* invaluable for the study and care of the patient with neuromuscular disease.

JAMES L. BENNINGTON, M.D.

PREFACE

The development in our understanding of muscle diseases has reached the stage when exact diagnosis in this field is no longer the prerequisite of a specialised muscle research centre. There is now an obligation in every advanced medical community to diagnose diseases of muscle as precisely as new knowledge and advancing techniques allow. The author has attempted to create a textbook of moderate size, concerned solely with muscle and neuromuscular diseases, and written with the main object of assisting in diagnosis. The existing textbooks, such as the three-volume compilation by G. H. Bourne, the work of many contributors edited by J. N. Walton, and the excellent book by R. D. Adams, D. Denny-Brown and C. M. Pearson, are all valuable reference publications but do not cater for the beginner in the subject or for general pathologists and general physicians who only occasionally encounter a difficult diagnostic problem in muscle disease.

This present book is based on an extensive experience of muscle diseases gained through the kindly interest of general physicians, paediatricians, and neurologists in the Oxford region. In the past 12 years a large number of biopsies and necropsies of cases of muscle diseases have been performed by members of the Department of Neuropathology at the Radcliffe Infirmary, Oxford. The author acknowledges with gratitude his indebtedness to his colleagues Dr. D. B. Brownell, Dr. D. R. Oppenheimer, and Dr. M. Esiri who have shared with him in the study of these cases, and to the numerous surgeons in the Oxford region and in particular to those of the Department of Neurological Surgery who have skillfully excised portions of muscle for biopsy.

For technical assistance I am indebted to Mr. R. A. Beesley and to successive members over many years of his technical staff. That part of the work involving electron microscopy has been ably supervised by Mr. D. Jerrome, and the electron micrographs have been prepared by Mrs. C. Forster and Mrs. K. Schomberg. The majority of the photomicrographs are the work of Dr. T. Parry. For assistance with references

I am grateful to Miss B. Newton and her staff of the Cairns Library at the Radcliffe Infirmary, Oxford, and to the staff of the Radcliffe Science Library, Oxford.

The manuscript was typed by Miss J. Mitchell and Mrs. J. Smith.

J. Trevor Hughes, M.D.

CONTENTS

Chapter One

Normal Muscle

Movement is one of the essential properties of a living organism and the few exceptions, notably the viruses, demonstrate the indistinct border between animate and inanimate things. Movement in most animals is made by cellular contractility; in a unicellular organism this is one of several functions of the single cell but in coelenterates it becomes a specialised function of certain surface epithelial cells. When we examine more complex animals we always find specialised muscle cells which contract to produce coordinated movements under the control of some type of nervous organisation (Clark, 1971).

In vertebrates the muscle cells are further specialised and three distinctive types of muscle may be recognised — *smooth, cardiac* and *striated* (the last named being also called *striped, somatic, skeletal* and *voluntary*). This monograph is concerned solely with human striated muscle and its disorders.

Our understanding of the morphology and function of striated muscle is much greater than our corresponding knowledge of smooth muscle and of cardiac muscle. While we cannot ignore known differences between these three fundamental muscle types, much of the information on the anatomical structure, on the physiology of contraction and on the biochemistry of action of muscle may prove relevant to all three forms of muscle.

EMBRYOLOGY

The development of human striated muscle in the embryonic (up to the end of the eighth week) and in the foetal (ninth week to term) period has been the subject of considerable research from which, apart from a few disputed areas, the majority of the facts have emerged. For reviews of the literature the reader is referred to Lewis (1910), Keith (1948), Starck (1955), Willis (1962) and Boyd (1960). Blechschmidt (1961) has

1

published an excellent atlas. In the account that follows, the subject will be divided into a description of the gross development of the body musculature followed by an account of the transformation of the primitive mesenchymal cell into the multinucleated striated muscle fibre.

Gross Development of Striated Muscle

All human striated muscle is derived from mesoderm, with the possible exception of the *sphincter pupillae,* which may, as has been shown in birds and reptiles, be ectodermal. There are, however, three different areas of mesoderm in which muscle arises: the myotomes of the somites, the branchial arches, and locally formed mesenchyme not derived from somites.

MUSCLE ARISING IN THE SOMITES

The muscle arising in the position of the embryonic somites (Fig. 1–1) is given prominence in many accounts, and in some (e.g., Adams, Denny-Brown and Pearson, 1962) this is the only source of muscle mentioned. This muscle is probably less in amount than that formed locally from mesenchyme. However the somites are so prominent in the embryo and their segmental origin so evident that we will describe this development first.

Two longitudinal bands of mesoderm, called the paraxial mesoderm, are developed on either side of the notochord. This paraxial mesoderm becomes segmented into somites, within which are the groups of cells differentiating towards muscle; these are called myotomes (Fig. 1–2). In the human embryo (Kunitomo, 1918) there are from 42 to 44 somites made up of 4 occipital, 8 cervical, 12 thoracic, 5 lumbar, 5 sacral and 8 to 10 coccygeal segments, and we can speak of similar named myotomes. The first occipital and most of the coccygeal somites disappear without giving rise to permanent structures. From the remaining three occipital myotomes are developed the tongue and the extrinsic muscles of the eye. The cervical myotomes give rise to the prevertebral and post-vertebral muscles of the neck. The posterior trunk musculature is derived from the thoracic and lumbar myotomes, but the lateral and anterior trunk muscles are probably not developed from myotomes.

MUSCLE ARISING IN THE BRANCHIAL ARCHES

The branchial arches (Fig. 1–1), which begin to appear during the fourth week, are a series of ridges (between which are furrows called the branchial grooves) on the ventro-lateral aspect of the embryonic head. In the human embryo there are five or six pairs of branchial arches;

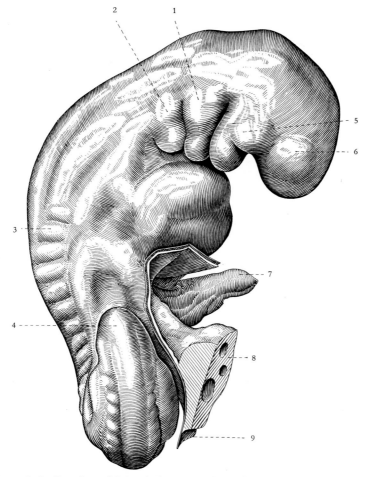

Figure 1–1 Drawing of 3.4 mm human embryo showing the development of the visceral arches and the somites: (1) second visceral arch; (2) third visceral arch; (3) second lateral segment; (4) coccyx; (5) maxillary bulge; (6) eye; (7) vitello-intestinal duct; (8) body stalk; (9) amnion. (From Blechschmidt, E.: The Stages of Human Development Before Birth. Karger & Saunders, 1961.)

these are considered to relate to the gill slits of lower vertebrates. The first branchial arch (mandibular) gives rise to the muscles of mastication, while the facial muscles are derived from the second (hyoid) arch. From the more caudal arches are developed the muscles of the pharynx and larynx.

MUSCLE ARISING FROM LOCALLY SITED MESODERM

It is now known that the greater part of the body musculature arises locally from non-somite mesenchyme. The muscles of the limbs and the majority of the trunk muscles are derived in this way. Lewis (1902) was

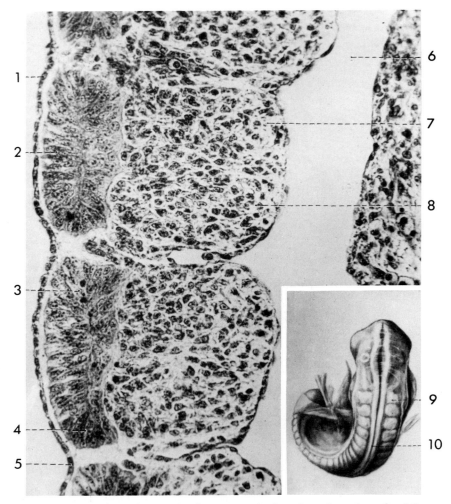

Figure 1-2 Photomicrograph of a para-sagittal section of somites of a 2.5 mm human embryo. (1) ectoderm; (2) sixth dermato-myotome; (3) upper growth area of dermato-myotome; (4) lower growth area of dermato-myotome; (5) intersegmental sulcus; (6) aorta; (7) and (8) sklerotome; (9) and (10) lateral segments. (From Blechschmidt, E.: The Stages of Human Development Before Birth. Karger & Saunders, 1961.)

convinced of this origin from his study of the development of the human arm muscles, and experimentally he showed (Lewis 1910) that excision of so-called "limb" myotomes in the embryonal stage of the salamander did not hinder the development of the limb muscles. In chick embryos, Straus and Rawles (1953) marked somites with carbon and showed that this did not enter the anterior and lateral trunk muscles, whereas this did occur when the lateral plate mesoderm was marked with carbon. In this way, the anterior and lateral trunk muscles were shown to arise from the outer part of the lateral plate mesoderm, which is immediately beneath the ectoderm and which is known as the somatopleuric meso-derm. The limb muscles arise *in situ* from the mesenchymal cells of the limb buds. These mesenchymal cells arise as collections of somato-pleuric cells near the coelomic epithelium and migrate towards the epidermis, which is then thrust out, enclosing this mesenchyme to form the limb bud. There is no subsequent contribution to these groups of mesenchyme cells from the myotomes of the somites. Probably not only the muscles but all of the connective tissues of the limbs are differ-entiated *in situ*.

Growth of Individual Muscles

In humans most of the muscle fibres appear to have been formed in the antenatal period (MacCallum, 1898); postnatal growth of a muscle is due to an increase in the length and diameter of the individual muscle fibres. The length of each sarcomere developed in foetal muscle is ap-proximately the same as that found in adult muscle, the muscle fibres of which may be up to 20 times as long. The increase in length of the muscle fibre appears to result from the addition of new sarcomeres to the end of the fibre; the increased diameter arises from an increase in the number of myofibrils, brought about by the splitting of other myofibrils and the formation of new myofibrils. At the same time as the enlargement of the muscle fibre there is an increase in the sarcoplasm and in the connective tissue and the vessels.

The growth of muscle is determined by several factors, of which the most important are the innervation and the state of muscle activity. Denervation slows muscle growth, but muscle still develops in the ab-sence of innervation. Muscle hypertrophies with activity and atrophies with inactivity. Atrophy can be demonstrated experimentally by using plaster casts to immobilise limbs or by severing the skeletal attachments of muscles. The hypertrophy induced by exercise depends on maximal isometric contraction of the muscle. Muscle growth is also controlled by hormones, and the varying output of these results in the growth spurts of adolescence. Muscle development in elderly persons can be stimu-lated by giving testosterone.

Development of the Striated Muscle Fibre

We now come to the stages in the transformation of the primitive mesenchymal cell into the multinucleate striated muscle fibre. The fol-lowing terms (Boyd, 1960) will be used for the successive stages in the differentiation of the muscle cell: *premyoblast, myoblast, myocyte, myotube* and *muscle fibre.* The older findings from light microscopy will be described first, and subsequently the additional information derived from electron microscopy. The primitive mesenchymal cells, which are destined to form muscle cells *(premyoblasts)*, can only be recognised as premyoblasts by their position when they arise as somato-pleuric cells near the coelomic epithelium. They are at this stage unremarkable, round or oval uninucleated or dividing cells with clear cytoplasm, and consequently are indistinguishable from the other rapidly dividing cells around them. Later these cells become more elongated and may be called *myoblasts*, although they still cannot be surely distinguished from fibroblasts. Mitotic figures are seen progressively less frequently when the cells are found to be elongated and have cytoplasmic granules. It is at this stage that the developing muscle cell becomes multinucleated.

Formation of the Multinucleated Muscle Cell

The premyoblast is a mononuclear cell, but some myoblasts and all of the later stages of the muscle cell are multinucleated. How this transition from a uninucleated to a multinucleated cell is brought about has been extensively studied, but the examination in histological sections of fixed embryonic material has not given conclusive results. In tissue cultures of myoblasts, fusion of cells has been repeatedly shown to occur (Okazaki and Holtzer, 1966). Yaffe and Feldman (1965) have in tissue culture fused rat myoblasts (labelled with tritiated thymidine) with unlabelled rabbit myoblasts. Mintz and Baker (1967) have approached the problem differently by joining two mouse blastomeres from parents having types of isocitrate dehydrogenase that differed electrophoretically. The resulting mouse muscle contained a hybrid enzyme. These experiments appear conclusive for tissue culture in which the multinucleated form arises largely by fusion. Probably the same method of formation occurs in the developing embryo. Mitotic figures seem to be rare at this stage of maturation and consequently the occurence of amitotic division has been suggested. However, amitotic division, though often postulated, has not been shown to be a common method of nuclear replication either in muscle or in other tissues.

The *myocyte* by development becomes the familiar *myotube* (Fig. 1-3), which is an elongated narrow cell with parallel borders and indistinct central cytoplasm. The numerous nuclei are central in position and the band structure is beginning to form. The contractile protein first appears as cytoplasmic granules which develop into the sarcomeres, and these arrange themselves into the familiar band striation.

From the *myotube* stage the mature muscle fibre develops further by elaboration of the contractile protein into myofibrils and the peripheral migration of the sarcolemmal nuclei. The stage of embryonic development at which these various maturing cells are evident cannot be stated

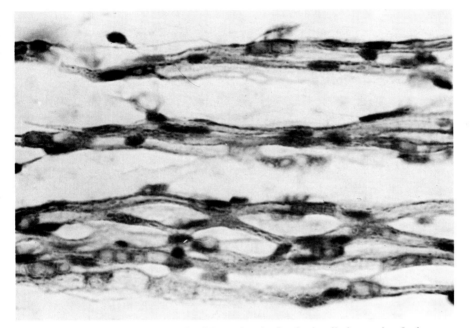

Figure 1-3   Photomicrograph of myotubes in developing limb muscle of a human foetus. (Haematoxylin and eosin, × 240).

concisely for all muscles, because muscle development proceeds earlier in the cephalad regions than in the caudal musculature.

The Ultrastructure of the Developing Muscle Fibre

The resolution possible with the electron microscope has provided important morphological details in our knowledge of muscle fibre development. The ultrastructural studies of Fischman (1967) suggest that the thin filaments (6 to 7 nm in thickness and up to 1.1 μm long) develop earlier than the thick filaments (16–17 nm wide and up to 1 μm long). Possibly thin filaments repel one another whereas thick and thin fibres are mutually attracted. The Z band (made up of tropomyosin) comes into existence because the actin filaments are arranged "back to back." When considering the formation of myofilaments it is of interest that Huxley (1963) has been able to form thick and thin filaments *in vitro* by the polymerisation of purified myosin and G-actin.

The sequence of growth of the structures making up the muscle fibre has been suggested by electron microscopical studies. The first myofibrils are formed immediately beneath the sarcolemma and each myofibril grows by the addition of myofilaments at its lateral margins. Myofibrils are said to divide longitudinally (Allbrook, 1962), but this is not certain, and subsequent myofibrils may form (as must the first) by the arrangement of myofilaments which are polymerised from large protein molecules.

The Role of the Satellite Cell

Mauro (1961) first observed in adult muscle cells discrete mononuclear cells situated between the basement membrane and the plasma membrane. Mauro and subsequent authors (MacConnachie, Enesco and Leblond, 1964) have considered that the satellite cell is the means of repair and replacement of damaged adult muscle fibres. In this light the satellite cell may be considered to be a resting myoblast, possessing the generative properties of myoblasts at an early stage of the development of the muscle fibre.

Development of Innervation of Muscle

With the light microscope Cuajunco (1942), examining human embryos at the tenth week, found nerve fibres near myotubules and, at the twelfth week, endings in contact with the muscle fibres. By the thirteenth week the nerve endings had penetrated the sarcolemma, and by the fourteenth week a mature nerve ending had formed. The ultrastructural studies of Filogamo and Gabella (1967) demonstrated fine nerve fibres in the myotomes of rat, rabbit and guinea pig embryos on the twelfth day after conception, and by the sixteenth day in the rat, terminal aborisations could be seen with silver staining and cholinesterase reaction showed activity near motor end-plates. The muscle spindle has been found to be innervated in the human foetus at the eleventh week, and its development appears to precede that of the motor end-plates (Cuajunco, 1940).

Development of the Muscle-Tendon Junctions

The development of the junction between muscle fibres and tendon fibres has been studied by Long (1947), who found both cells developed simultaneously but not in continuity. Muir (1961) has shown with the electron microscope that during development the end of the muscle fibre has sarcolemmal invaginations into which are inserted prolongations of the tendon collagen.

MACROSCOPICAL ANATOMY

The skeletal muscles form about 40 per cent of the weight of the human adult and their activity accounts for a substantial proportion of the metabolic requirements of the body. There are over 400 individually named muscles of varying size and function. These muscles range from the gluteus maximus, which is the largest, to the muscle tensing the human eardrum, which is the smallest. Between these two extremes are muscles of varying size and power, differing also in their speed and range of movement. Human muscles differ not only in the size of their muscle bellies but also in the size of the fibres making up the individual muscles. In general the small muscles have small fibres and the large muscles have large fibres.

The length of muscle fibres is difficult to ascertain in histological sections, but has been estimated by teasing out individual fibres, which are obtained singly by partial maceration in weak alkali solutions. Muscle fibres are long in long muscles such as the sartorius muscle and short in short muscles such as the extrinsic muscles of the eye. Most individual muscles have two points of attachment, usually to bone, but there seems always to be an intervening tendon between a muscle and its attachment. A muscle belly may have various arrangements of its muscle fibres. If the muscle fibres converge into a single tendon, the muscle is said to be *unipennate*, and if this arrangement is found at both ends of the muscle, the muscle is said to be *bipennate*. Compound muscles, which have several bellies, are said to be *multipennate*.

It is appropriate here to make a few remarks about muscle actions, which were classified by Beevor (1904). A *prime mover* is a muscle acting directly on its insertion in its principal function. Muscles never act alone, and the ancillary action of another muscle supporting or modifying the action of the prime mover classifies such a muscle as either a *synergist* or an *antagonist*. When a muscle contracts fully there is shortening to about 50 per cent of its original length. This action, during which the tone of the muscle may remain the same, is called *isotonic contraction*. A muscle may also act by causing tension without shortening, and muscles often exert their greatest power in this way. This type of contraction, when there is an increase in tension without shortening, is called *isometric contraction*.

MICROSCOPICAL ANATOMY

Every muscle belly is surrounded by a connective tissue sheath, called the *epimysium* (Fig. 1–4). From this outer epimysium, fibrous septa pass inward and divide the muscle into compartments containing large numbers of muscle fibres. These intramuscular connective tissue septa and the sheaths which they form around bundles of muscle fibres constitute the *perimysium* (Fig. 1–5). From the perimysium are derived thinner strands of connective tissue which separate the individual muscle fibres and enclose each fibre in a fine connective tissue sheath called the *endomysium*.

These connective tissue layers consist of collagen fibres together

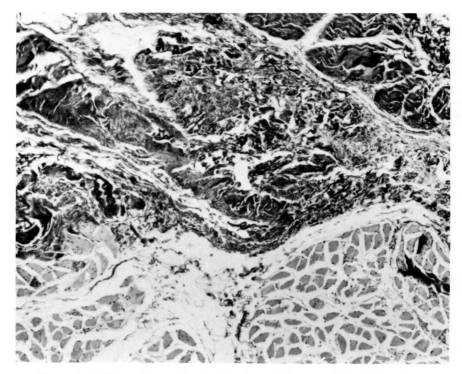

Figure 1–4 Photomicrograph of epimysium. Only part of the thick collagenous sheath is shown in the picture. (Haematoxylin and eosin, × 25.)

with some reticulum fibres and elastic fibres. The cells concerned are mainly fibroblasts, but there are also fat cells and histiocytes. The amount of connective tissue in a muscle and the pattern of the connective tissue matrix is determined by the function of the muscle; the connective tissue makes an important contribution towards the tension of a muscle, particularly when the muscle is at rest. Muscles are connected to their final attachments by intervening tendons, and the anatomy of the junction between the muscle fibre and the tendon fibre has been extensively studied. It was thought that the cytoplasm of the muscle fibre was actually continuous with that of the tendon fibre, but this seems not to be the case. There is probably a connective tissue attachment between the endomysium of the muscle fibre and the basement membrane of the tendon cell.

The light microscopical appearance of the striated muscle fibre has been studied for several centuries. This remarkable cell is a large multinucleated cell which in human muscle varies in width from 10 to 100 μm and in length from 1 to 15 cm. The measurements of length are an average, and in some muscles, such as the human sartorius, Lockhart and Brandt (1938) found muscle fibres up to a length of 34 cm. It is still

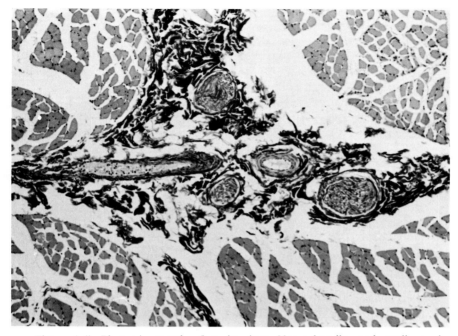

Figure 1–5 Photomicrograph of perimysium. Nerve bundles and small vessels can be seen among the connective tissue separating the fascicles of muscle fibres. (Haematoxylin and eosin, × 25.)

not certain whether these long muscle fibres are entirely continuous or are made up of shorter cells linked at their ends.

The muscle fibre is a multinucleated syncytium and the nuclei, which may number up to 200, are situated at the periphery of the cell, immediately beneath the sarcolemmal sheath. There is no recognisable arrangement by which the cytoplasm is under the influence of any nucleus or nuclei, and the manner in which the function of the cell is co-ordinated is not known. In longitudinal and in transverse sections it can be readily seen that the muscle fibre is divided into large numbers of longitudinal strands called myofibrils. These myofibrils are approximately 1 μm in diameter, and up to 100 myofibrils may be present within a single muscle fibre. These myofibrils are considered to be within a matrix called the sarcoplasm. The detailed structure of the muscle fibre will be considered later, in the light of modern ultramicroscopic observations.

The transverse striated appearance of the skeletal muscle fibre, from which is derived the name of striated or striped muscle, is evident in many staining techniques and can also be seen in unstained sections. We know now from electron microscopy that the striation is due to the arrangement of the myofilaments in the myofibril, and, because adjacent myofibrils have the same instep arrangement of myofilaments, that the transverse banding goes across the whole muscle fibre and gives the striped appearance. Even with light microscopy these striations were already sufficiently well documented for the banding to have special names. Originally the banding was recognised as an alternation of dark bands and light bands. The dark bands were called the A bands (anisotrophic) because they were strongly birefringent when viewed with polarised light. The intervening light bands were called the I bands (isotrophic) because they were not birefringent. Two thin lines, one light in shade in the middle of the dark A band, and one dark in shade in the middle of the light I band, had also been recognised. The light line in the middle of the A band is known as the M line (Mittelschiebe) and the dark line in the middle of the light line is known as the Z line (Zwischenschiebe).

ULTRASTRUCTURE

The use of the electron microscope in conjunction with modern techniques of ultrathin section-cutting has greatly increased our understanding of the anatomy of biological tissues. One example of this is our knowledge of the ultrastructure of muscle fibres. For reviews of this the reader is referred to Bennett (1960), Huxley (1960), Huxley and Hanson (1960), and Price (1969).

The ultrastructure of the muscle fibre will be considered under the following headings: *sarcolemmal nuclei, sarcolemma, band structure, tubular system organelles,* and *miscellaneous particles.*

SARCOLEMMAL NUCLEI

The large ovoid elongated nuclei situated peripherally under the sarcolemma have an unremarkable ultrastructural appearance (Fig. 1–6), presumably because the morphological features of the nucleus that might reveal details of its function are only evident during mitosis. The nucleus is contained in a double-layered membrane, and apertures (pores) in the outer membrane communicate with the sarcoplasmic reticulum of the muscle cell.

SARCOLEMMA

There is some confusion in terminology, but here the convention is followed that the sarcolemma consists of the double-layered sheath which invests an individual muscle fibre. It has an outer basement membrane and an inner plasma membrane (Fig. 1–6). The thick basement membrane, reinforced on the outside with scattered collagen

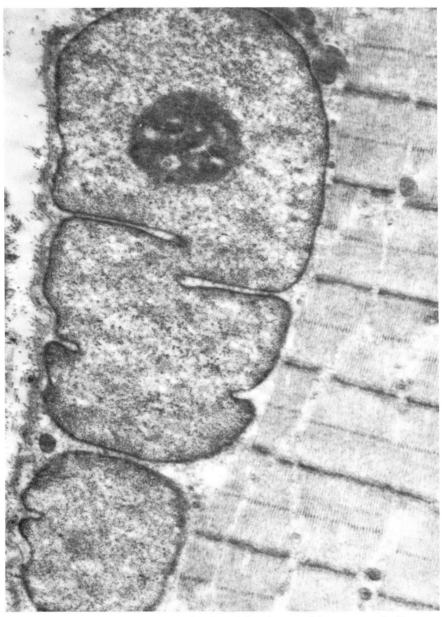

Figure 1–6 Electron micrograph of peripheral part of human muscle fibre cut longitudinally. The sarcolemmal nucleus has a prominent nucleolus. Note the double-layered membrane surrounding the nucleus and the two layers of the sarcolemma. (Phosphotungstic acid, × 14,000.)

fibres, constitutes the main supportive and protective membrane of the mature muscle fibre. It remains intact after damage to the fibre, and regeneration may then occur within the empty tube. It appears not to atrophy when the muscle cell shrinks from denervation. The basement membrane of the muscle fibre is an unusual structure in biology, and similar sheaths are found in relation to only a few other mammalian cells. The basement membrane is not present around the myoblasts of foetal muscle nor around regenerating muscle fibres. The plasma membrane is a thin (approximately 7.5 nm), triple-layered membrane closely investing the muscle cell and having the same structure and function as the plasma membrane of other cells. When the muscle fibre atrophies the plasma membrane shrinks.

BAND STRUCTURE

One benefit from the application to biology of the electron microscope was the elucidation of the nature of the band structure of striated muscle. The myofibril was found to be made up of myofilaments consisting of a double array of interdigitating thick and thin filaments. The thick filaments (15 to 17 nm in diameter) make up the A band to a degree that depends on the amount of contraction of the muscle fibre. The thick filaments are made up of myosin molecules. The thin filaments (5 to 6 nm in diameter) form the I band and are made up of actin molecules. The Z line, where the thin filaments are connected, appears to contain tropomyosin, a third specialised muscle protein.

The arrangement of myofilaments just described can be readily seen in ultrathin sections cut in the longitudinal plane of the muscle fibre (Fig. 1–7). In similarly prepared transverse sections the myofibrils appear as hexagonal areas in which the transversely cut myofilaments appear as dots. If the section passes through the A band, the dots are of the thick myosin filaments. If the section passes through the I band the dots are of small diameter actin filaments. Between the centre and the margin of the sarcomere, and to a degree that would depend on the state of contraction, the transverse section would cut a mixture of thick and thin myofilaments.

TUBULAR SYSTEM

Muscle appears to have two independent tubular networks: the sarcoplasmatic reticulum and the transverse tubular system (T-system). They are not thought to communicate with one another. The *sarcoplasmic reticulum* appears to be analogous to the endoplasmic reticulum found in other cells, and does not appear to connect with the extracellular space. It consists of an extensive network of small diameter tubular channels which often expand into larger sacs, the whole network ramifying around the myofibrils. The *transverse tubular system* (T-system) con-

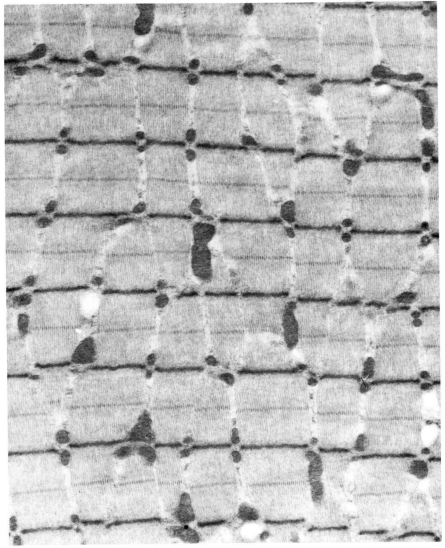

Figure 1-7   Electron micrograph of central part of human muscle fibre cut longitudinally. About seven myofibrils can be seen and between them lie the mitochondria and elements of the tubular system. (Phosphotungstic acid, × 14,000.)

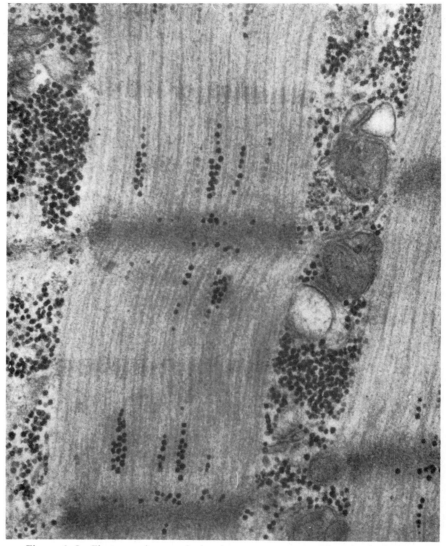

Figure 1–8   Electron micrograph showing two sarcomeres. Note the dark glycogen granules, the mitochondria, and the two components of the tubular system. (2% aqueous uranyl acetate and lead citrate, × 50,000.)

sists of smaller tubular channels that do not expand into big cisterns. These channels also surround the myofibrils as a network. The transverse tubular system comes into regular relationship with the sarcoplasmic reticulum to form the triads (Fig. 1–8). These *triads*, which are situated at the junction of the A and I bands, are made up of a central channel of the T-system between two cisterns of the sarcoplasmic reticulum.

ORGANELLES

The organelles recognised in the muscle cell are the mitochondria, the Golgi complex and the lysosomes.

Mitochondria, which are present in nearly all animal cells, are of great importance in metabolism; for a general account of their structure and function the reader is referred to the reviews of Novikoff (1961) and of Lehninger (1964). In human muscle fibres, mitochondria are abundant, particularly in type I fibres, where they are prominent in the intermyofibrillar regions (Fig. 1–8); in the subsarcolemmal region; and around the sarcolemmal nuclei. They have not been shown to differ in structure from the mitochondria of other cells, and the variety in size and shape of mitochondria that may be found cannot yet be correlated to any difference in the activity of the muscle fibre. Degeneration of mitochondria is often observed; this must be distingushed from artefact changes, which are common with glutaraldehyde fixation. Inclusions are sometimes present within mitochondria, the commonest being electron dense granules. Glycogen granules and lipid granules may also be present within mitochondria.

The *Golgi complex* (Price, 1963) is not well seen in adult muscle fibres. It appears as a system of flattened tubular channels situated in the cell cytoplasm near either the upper or the lower pole of the sarcolemmal nucleus. It is more conspicuous in developing muscle fibres and in muscle fibres undergoing regeneration. For a general review of the structure and function of the Golgi apparatus the reader is referred to Dalton (1961). Information is still lacking concerning the importance of this organelle in the growth and activity of the muscle fibre.

In common with most other animal cells, muscle fibres contain *lysosomes*, the membrane-bound digestive chambers rich in acid hydrolases discovered by de Duve at the University of Louvain in 1949. For a general account of this important structure the reader is referred to Dingle and Fell (1969). Lysosomes are now known to be present in small numbers in normal human muscle (Fig. 1–9). They are prominent in many states of degeneration of muscle and are also seen in the atrophying process of muscle undergoing denervation. Detailed evidence of the action of acid hydrolases within lysosomes in the loss of the muscle constituents from an atrophying muscle fibre is presented by Weinstock and Iodice (1969). In studying human diseases by the electron micros-

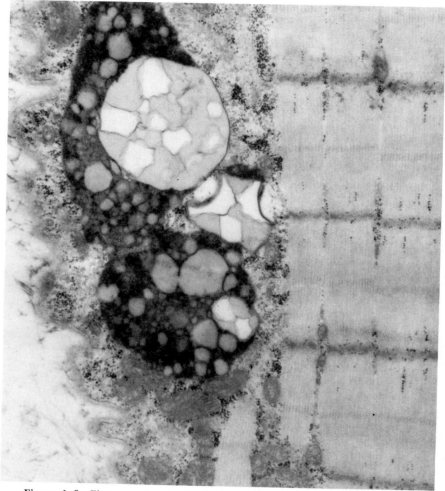

Figure 1-9 Electron micrograph showing edge of human muscle fibre cut longitudinally. The structure shown is a membrane-bound digestive chamber called a lysosome. This may be seen, as here, in a normal muscle fibre, but is common in most degenerating muscle fibres. (2% aqueous uranyl acetate and lead citrate, × 20,000.)

copy of excised portions of muscle, lysosomes are readily seen beneath the sarcolemma and often conspicuously around sarcolemmal nuclei in the centre of the muscle fibre.

MISCELLANEOUS PARTICLES

Glycogen granules, measuring from 25 to 40 nm in diameter and staining intensely with lead, are prominent throughout muscle fibres, but probably vary according to the nutritional and metabolic activity at the time the muscle is examined. Glycogen granules are most conspicuous immediately beneath the sarcolemma and in the interfibrillar spaces (Fig. 1–8), but they may also be seen between individual myofilaments. Glycogen is more plentiful in the type II muscle fibre and is increased in some of the metabolic diseases of muscle.

Lipid particles, appearing as medium-sized round bodies with a homogenous content of material of medium electron density, are present in normal human muscle and are common in certain myopathic conditions (Fig. 1–10). In normal muscle they are commonly found among

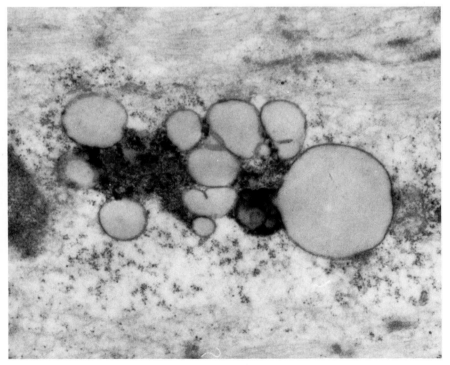

Figure 1–10   Electron micrograph showing lipid particles in centre of a degenerating human muscle fibre. These particles may coalesce to form a lysosome. (2% aqueous uranyl acetate and lead citrate, × 26,400.)

mitochondria, either beneath the sarcolemma or in the intermyofibrillar spaces. They are commoner in the type I (granular) fibres.

Lipofuchsin material is frequently identified in human muscle and sometimes may not be distinguishable from lysosomes. Lipofuchsin is found in irregular aggregates which frequently include lipid droplets.

Ribosomes are seen in muscle as very small (15 nm) electron-dense particles, in clusters or arranged along fine membranes or filaments. They are presumed to be concerned with protein synthesis but their function in muscle has not been specifically studied.

INNERVATION

The region of a muscle where the nerve supply (and the blood supply) enters may be sufficiently well defined as to merit the term *neurovascular hilum*. Brash (1955) has compiled an atlas of the neurovascular hila of the limb muscles. There are two main types of neurovascular hila: the interfascicular, in which the nerves enter parallel to the muscle bundles of long muscles (e.g., sartorius), and the transfascicular, where the nerve trunks proceed in a direction transverse to the muscle bundles (e.g., gluteus maximus). A complex muscle may have several points where nerve trunks enter, particularly if, as in the rectus abdominus muscle, the innervation is derived in a segmental manner from

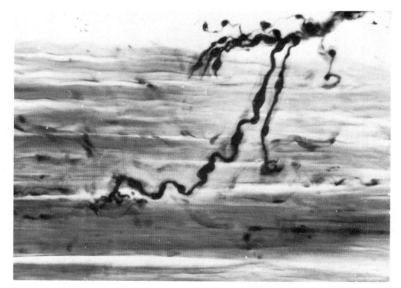

Figure 1–11 Human muscle stained by a silver technique to show axons. The photomicrograph shows the final branching of a motor nerve. (Schofield's technique, × 160.)

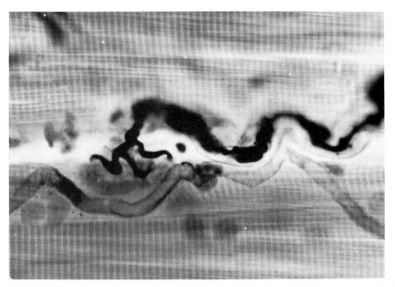

Figure 1–12 Photomicrograph at higher magnification of the motor end plate seen in Figure 1–11. (Schofield's technique, × 500.)

several consecutive spinal cord segments. The nerve fibres contained in a "motor" nerve will be a mixture of efferent and afferent fibres, with efferent fibres forming rather more than 50 per cent. Most of the nerve fibres are myelinated. The *efferent* nerve fibres arise as the axons of anterior horn neurone cell bodies. An individual axon divides probably within the peripheral nerve trunk and certainly within the muscle, so that 10 to 100 branches are formed (Fig. 1–11), each of which terminates on one muscle fibre in a structure known as a motor end-plate (Fig. 1–12). The anterior horn perikaryon, its main axon and all the nerve branches, together with the group of muscle fibres which they supply, constitute a *motor unit*. The number of muscle fibres forming a motor unit is small in muscles of fine movement (e.g., extrinsic eye muscles, lumbricals) and large in muscles of grosser movement (proximal limb muscles). Near its termination, the efferent nerve fibre loses its myelin sheath, after which there is a final branching into the axonic processes of the motor end-plate (Fig. 1–12). These terminal branches are unmyelinated but have a thin connective tissue sheath derived from modified Schwann cells (called teloglia by Couteaux, 1960).

The terminal arborisation of the motor end-plate consists of expansions of axoplasm containing synaptic vesicles rich in cholinesterase activity. For a detailed review of the structure of the motor end-plate the reader is referred to Coërs and Woolf (1959), Couteaux (1960) and Zacks (1964).

The *afferent fibres* from the muscles arise either from simple unbranched terminals applied to the outside of the muscle fibres or from the complex sensory organs called muscle spindles. The first type are often called *free nerve endings*. They are not well understood but are usually considered to be fine fibres involved in pain sensation. Some are well seen around blood vessels and form part of the autonomic nervous system. The specialised muscle sensory receptors called muscle spindles have an extensive innervation that has received a great deal of study, much of which is detailed in the reviews of Cuajunco (1940), Barker (1948), Cooper (1960), and Barker (1962).

Muscle spindles are present in all voluntary muscles, but their size and number vary. A muscle spindle consists of a fusiform connective tissue sac in which are contained several specialised muscle fibres called intrafusal muscle fibres (Fig. 1–13). The muscle spindle has a motor innervation in which each intrafusal muscle fibre bears two motor end-plates (Barker, 1948). There are two afferent nerve fibre systems originally distinguished as primary and secondary by Ruffini (1898), whose observations have been confirmed by modern observers (Fig. 1–14).

In addition to the afferent nerve fibres arising from the free nerve endings and the muscle spindles, a "motor" nerve will also have nerve fibres arising from Golgi tendon organs and from Golgi-Mazzoni corpuscles, both of which are specialised stretch receptors related to tendon. Such nerve fibres may accompany other intramuscular nerve fibres to join the complement of nerve fibres within the motor nerve.

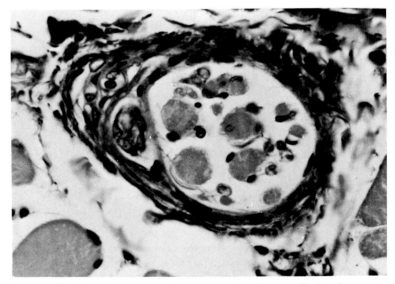

Figure 1–13   Muscle spindle in human muscle. The spindle has been cut transversely somewhere near the equatorial region. Note the small intrafusal muscle fibres and the nerve within the connective tissue compartment on the left. (Haematoxylin and van Gieson, × 500.)

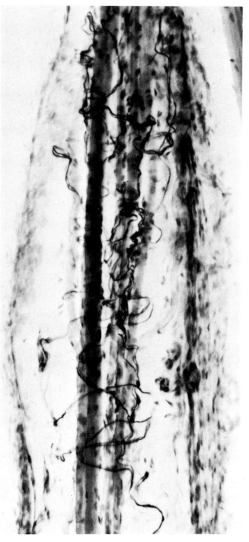

Figure 1-14 Human muscle spindle. The photomicrograph shows part of the complicated innervation of the spindle as seen in a longitudinal section stained for nerve axons. (Schofield's technique, × 170.)

BLOOD SUPPLY

The blood supply of voluntary muscle has not received much recent attention, and for a review the reader is referred to Walls (1960). Voluntary muscle requires a rich blood supply to sustain its enormous metabolism. The larger muscular arteries enter at definite neuromuscular hila (Brash, 1955) and in their major branches accompany the nerve trunks. These major arterial divisions ramify in the perimysium (Figs. 1–15 and 1–16) but despite the apparent richness of this arterial plexus, intramuscular anastomosis appears inadequate to withstand occlusion of a major arterial trunk. (Clark and Blomfield, 1945). From the arterial plexus in the perimysium arise the smaller arteries, which lie transverse to the direction of the muscle fibres and give rise to the capillaries that run longitudinally between the muscle fibres (Figs. 1–17 and 1–18). The capillary plexus in the endomysium is particularly large; two or more transverse linking branches, when uniting two parallel capillaries separated by a muscle fibre, give rise to striking capillary rectangles. In addition to these data about the morphological appearance of the blood vessels supplying muscle, it is clearly of great importance that the blood supply of muscle will increase very substantially during exercise. Measurements and calculations on this potential reserve of blood supply were made on a variety of animals by Krogh (1919, 1922).

The *lymphatic vessels* within muscle appear to be confined to the perimysium and epimysium, although in the studies by injection techniques small lymph spaces have also been seen around individual muscle fibres. Lymph follicles do not appear to be present within skeletal muscle.

HISTOCHEMISTRY

The application of histochemical techniques to skeletal muscle has been helpful in the understanding of the biochemical reactions of developing and mature muscle, in the identification of two major histochemical types of muscle fibre, and in the demonstration of certain metabolic diseases caused by a specific enzyme deficiency. The subject has grown to very large proportions and will not be dealt with in detail here. The reader is referred to the following reviews: Beckett and Bourne (1960), Engel (1962), Dubowitz (1965, 1966, 1969) and Pearse (1968). A companion volume to this publication will present a detailed account of histochemistry as applied to human voluntary muscle.

Most of the histochemical techniques applicable to muscle are methods of demonstrating a specific enzyme. Over 50 enzyme systems can now be recognised and assessed in muscle but in most laboratories only a few of these would be justified in the routine examination of a muscle biopsy (Figs. 1–19, 1–20, and 1–21). In this author's laboratory
(*Text continued on page 28.*)

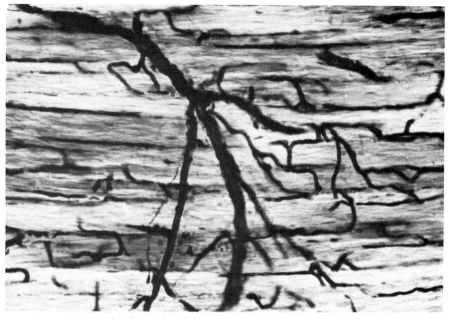

Figure 1–15 Blood supply of human muscle. The photomicrograph shows the final branching of a small muscle artery. (Schofield's technique, × 200.)

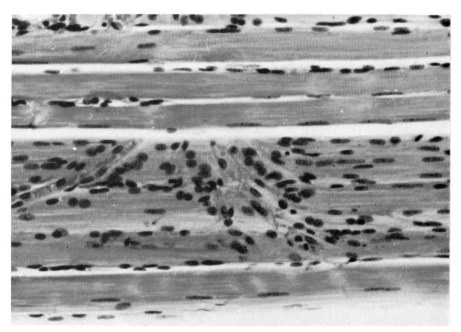

Figure 1–16 Photomicrograph comparable to Figure 1–15 as seen in a conventional stain. The great extent of the vascular supply is not so apparent here. (Haematoxylin and eosin, × 200.)

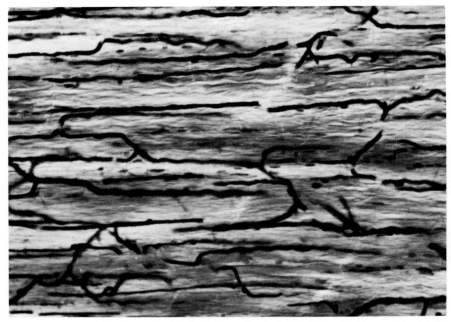

Figure 1–17   Arcades of capillaries between individual muscle fibres. (Schofield's technique, × 200.)

Figure 1–18   Photomicrograph comparable to Figure 1–17 but showing histological structure as seen in a conventional stain. (Haematoxylin and eosin, × 200.)

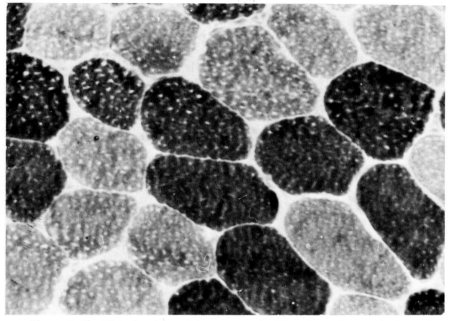

Figure 1-19 Histochemistry of human muscle. The photomicrograph shows the adenosine triphosphatase (ATP-ase) reaction on normal muscle. Only half the muscle fibres show a positive reaction. (ATP-ase reaction, × 250.)

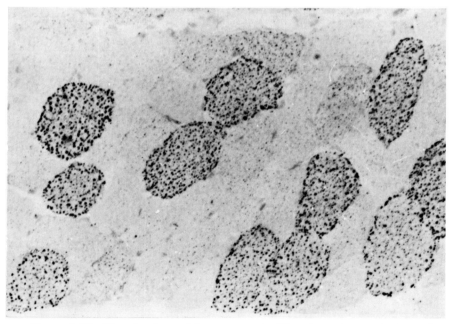

Figure 1-20 Histochemistry of human muscle. The photomicrograph shows the succinic dehydrogenase reaction (SDH-ase) on normal muscle. Only half the muscle fibres show a positive reaction. (SDH-ase reaction, × 250.)

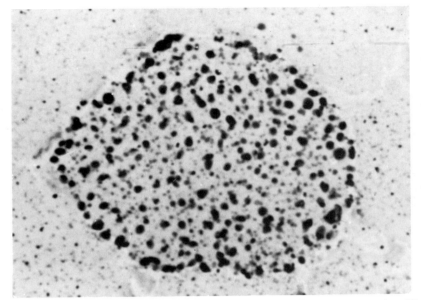

Figure 1–21   Detail of SDH-ase positive muscle fibre cut in transverse section. The enzyme activity is centered in the mitochondria, which appear as dark dots. (SDH-ase reaction, × 1000.)

the following enzyme reactions are regularly used: *myofibrillar adenosine triphosphatase* (ATP-ase), *phosphorylase,* and *succinic dehydrogenase* (SDH-ase). These enzyme reactions serve to differentiate granular (type I) from agranular (type II) muscle fibres, since ATP-ase and phosphory-lase are largely present in type II fibre and SDH-ase in type I fibres.

In addition to the demonstration of muscle enzymes, certain other histochemical procedures are of value in the examination of muscle. The *periodic acid–Schiff reaction* is valuable mainly because, together with other tests, it can determine the amount of glycogen in the muscle. Neutral fat can be demonstrated by the use of Sudan black or of oil-red-0 on frozen sections.

BIOCHEMISTRY

Space does not allow more than a list of the chemical constituents of striated muscle and a mere mention of the principal biochemical reactions that have been discovered. Of the many reviews on this subject the following are recommended: Szent-Györgyi (1948, 1950, 1953), Mommaerts (1950), Adams, Denny-Brown and Pearson (1962), Gergely (1969) and Pennington (1969).

The chemical constituents of a striated muscle fibre may be considered under the following headings: *contractile proteins, myoglobin, enzymes, carbohydrates, lipids, nitrogenous compounds,* and *electrolytes.*

CONTRACTILE PROTEINS

The three main components of the contractile mechanism of muscle are myosin, actin and tropomyosin; these, together with myoglobin, make up the bulk of the protein within the muscle fibre. Myoglobin is the iron-bound protein which has a similar structure to the haemoglobin of red blood cells. It contributes to the red colour of muscle and is present in greater amounts in the "red" muscles of certain animals which have muscles specialised for prolonged contraction. In human muscle the muscle fibres appear to be a mixture of the two main biochemical types; the granular (type I) human muscle fibres are similar to the muscle fibres making up a "red" muscle in animals.

MUSCLE ENZYMES

The study of these now forms a very large subject which includes many of the biochemical processes common to all mammalian cells. The subject has been mentioned in the preceding section on histochemistry and will be referred to in describing the metabolic diseases of muscle.

CARBOHYDRATES

The various carbohydrates present in muscle are glycogen, glucose, and the various compounds forming the intermediary steps in the degeneration of glycogen to pyruvates and lactates. Muscle glycogen appears to be formed within the muscle from glucose and is an important method of energy storage.

LIPIDS

The lipids that can be extracted from muscle include *phospholipids, cholesterol, free fatty acids* and *triglycerides.* These fatty substances are known to be present in normal muscle, but their role in metabolism is not clear.

NITROGENOUS COMPOUNDS

A variety of nitrogenous compounds are present in muscle. There are many amino acids concerned with protein metabolism and of these, creatine is present in the greatest amount. The other group of non-protein nitrogen compounds are the *nucleotides,* chiefly *adenosine triphosphatide.*

ELECTROLYTES

The electrolytes present within muscle fibres differ markedly in their concentration from the levels of these constituents in blood plasma and in the extracellular fluid. Potassium is present in large amounts compared with the levels in the plasma. Phosphorous, magnesium and calcium are present, while the chief anion is chloride. Clearly the electrolyte concentrations within the muscle fibre are of the utmost importance in understanding its metabolism, and in particular the complex biochemistry of the contraction of muscle.

References

Adams, R. D., Denny-Brown, D., and Pearson, C. M. (1962). Diseases of Muscle. 2nd ed. Kimpton, London.

Allbrook, D. (1962). An electron microscopic study of regenerating skeletal muscle. J. Anat. *96*, 137–152.

Barker, D. (1948). The innervation of the muscle-spindle. Quart. J. Micro. Sci. *89*, 143–186.

Barker, D. (1962). Symposium on muscle receptors. Hong Kong University Press, Hong Kong.

Beckett, E. B., and Bourne, G. H. (1960). Histochemistry of skeletal muscle and changes in some muscle diseases. Chapter 9 *in* The Structure and Function of Muscle, Vol. III. G. H. Bourne (Ed.). Academic Press, New York & London.

Beevor, C. E. (1904). Croonian lectures on muscular movements. Adlard and Son, London.

Bennett, H. S. (1960). The structure of striated muscle as seen by the electron microscope. Chapter 6 *in* The Structure and Function of Muscle, Vol. I. G. H. Bourne (Ed.). Academic Press, New York & London.

Blechschmidt, E. (1961). The Stages of Human Development Before Birth. W. B. Saunders Company, Philadelphia & London.

Boyd, J. D. (1960). Development of striated muscle. Chapter 3 *in* The Structure and Function of Muscle, Vol. I. G. H. Bourne (Ed.). Academic Press. New York & London.

Brash, J. C. (1955). Neurovascular hila of limb muscles. Livingstone, Edinburgh & London.

Clark, W. E. LeG. (1971). The Tissues of the Body. 6th ed. Clarendon Press, Oxford.

Clark, W. E. LeG., and Blomfield, L. B. (1945). The efficiency of intramuscular anastomoses, with observations on the regeneration of devascularized muscle. J. Anat. *79*, 15–32.

Coërs, C., and Woolf, A. L. (1959). The Innervation of Muscle: A Biopsy Study. Charles C Thomas, Springfield, Illinois.

Cooper, S. (1960). Muscle spindles and other muscle receptors. Chapter 11 *in* The Structure and Function of Muscle, Vol. I. G. H. Bourne (Ed.). Academic Press, New York & London.

Couteaux, R. (1960). Motor end-plate structure. Chapter 10 *in* The Structure and Function of Muscle, Vol. I. G. H. Bourne (Ed.). Academic Press, New York & London.

Cuajunco, F. (1940). Development of the neuromuscular spindle in human fetuses. Carnegie Inst. Wash. Publ. 518. Contrib. Embryol. *28*, 98–128.

Cuajunco, F. (1942). Development of the motor end plate. Carnegie Inst. Wash. Contrib. Embryol. *30*, 127.

Dalton, A. J. (1961). Golgi apparatus and secretion granules. Chapter 8 *in* The Cell, Vol. II. J. Brachet and A. E. Mirsky (Eds.). Academic Press, New York & London.

Dingle, J. T., and Fell, H. B. (1969). Lysosomes in Biology and Pathology. North Holland Publishing Co., Amsterdam & London.

Dubowitz, V. (1965). Enzyme histochemistry of skeletal muscle. I. Developing animal muscle. II. Developing human muscle. J. Neurol. Neurosurg. Psychiat. *28*, 516–524.

Dubowitz, V. (1966). Enzyme histochemistry of skeletal muscle. III. Neurogenic muscular atrophies. J. Neurol. Neurosurg. Psychiat. *29*, 23–28.

Dubowtiz, V. (1969). Histochemical aspects of muscle disease. Chapter 8 *in* Disorders of Voluntary Muscle, 2nd ed. J. N. Walton (Ed.). Churchill, London.

Engel, W. K. (1962). The essentiality of histo- and cytochemical studies of skeletal muscle in the investigation of neuromuscular disease. Neurology (Minneap.) *12*, 778–794.

Filogamo, G., and Gabella, G. (1967). The development of neuromuscular correlations in vertebrates. Arch. Biol. *78*, 9–60.

Fischman, D. A. (1967). An electron microscope study of myofibril formation in embryonic chick skeletal muscle. J. Cell. Biol. *32*, 557–575.

Gergely, J. (1969). Biochemical aspects of muscular structure and function. *In* Disorders of Voluntary Muscle. 2nd ed. J. N. Walton (Ed.). Churchill, London.

Huxley, H. E. (1960). Muscle cells. Chapter 7 *in* The Cell, Vol. IV. J. Brachet and A. E. Mirsky (Eds.). Academic Press, New York & London.

Huxley, H. E. (1963). Electron microscope studies of natural and synthetic protein filaments from striated muscle. J. Mol. Biol. *7*, 281–308.

Huxley, H. E., and Hanson, J. (1960). The molecular basis of contraction in cross-striated muscles. Chapter 7 *in* The Structure and Function of Muscle, Vol. I. G. H. Bourne (Ed.). Academic Press, New York & London.

Keith, A. (1948). Human Embryology and Morphology. 6th ed. Arnold, London.

Krogh, A. (1919). The number and distribution of capillaries in muscle with calculations of the oxygen pressure head necessary for supplying the tissue. J. Physiol. (London) *52*, 409–415.

Krogh, A. (1922). The Anatomy and Physiology of Capillaries. Yale University Press, New Haven.

Kunitomo, K. (1918). The development and reduction of the tail and of the caudal end of the spinal cord. Carnegie Inst. Wash. Contrib. Embryol. *8*, 161–198.

Lehninger, A. L. (1964). The Mitochondrion: Molecular Basis of Structure and Function. W. A. Benjamin, New York.

Lewis, W. H. (1902). The development of the arm in man. Amer. J. Anat. *1*, 145–184.

Lewis, W. H. (1910). The development of the muscular system. *In* Keibel and Mall: Manual of Human Embryology, Vol. I, pp. 454–522. Lippincott, Philadelphia.

Lockhart, R. D., and Brandt, W. (1938). Length of striated muscle fibre. J. Anat. *72*, 470.

Long, M. E. (1947). Development of muscle-tendon attachment in rat. Amer. J. Anat. *81*, 159–197.

MacCallum, J. B. (1898). On the histogenesis of the striated muscle and the growth of the human sartorius muscle. Johns Hopkins Hosp. Bull. *9*, 208–215.

MacConnachie, H. F., Enesco, M., and Leblond, C. P. (1964). The mode of increase in the number of skeletal muscle nuclei in the postnatal rat. Amer. J. Anat. *114*, 245–253.

Mauro, A. (1961). Satellite cell of skeletal muscle fibres. J. Biophys. Biochem. Cytol. *9*, 493–495.

Mintz, B., and Baker, W. W. (1967). Normal mammalian muscle differentiation and gene control of isocitrate dehydrogenase synthesis. Proc. Nat. Acad. Sci. (U.S.A.) *58*, 592–598.

Mommaerts, W. F. H. M. (1950). Muscular Contraction. Interscience Publishers, New York & London.

Muir, A. R. (1961). Observations on the attachment of myofibrils to the sarcolemma at the muscle-tendon junction. *In* Electron Microscopy in Anatomy. J. D. Boyd, F. R. Johnson and J. D. Lever (Eds.). Arnold, London.

Novikoff, A. B. (1961). Mitochondria (chondriosomes). *In* The Cell. J. Brachet and A. E. Mirsky (Eds.). Academic Press, New York & London.

Okazaki, K., and Holtzer, H. (1966). Myogenesis: fusion, myosin synthesis and the mitotic cycle. Proc. Nat. Acad. Sci. (U.S.A.) *56*, 1484–1490.

Pearse, A. G. E. (1968). Histochemistry, Theoretical and Applied. 3rd ed. Churchill, London.

Pennington, R. J. T. (1969). Biochemical aspects of muscle disease. *In* Disorders of Voluntary Muscle. J. N. Walton (Ed.). Churchill, London.

Price, H. M. (1963). The skeletal muscle fibre in the light of electron microscope studies. Amer. J. Med. *35*, 589–605.

Price, H. M. (1969). Ultrastructure of the skeletal muscle fibre. *In* Disorders of Voluntary Muscle. J. N. Walton (Ed.). Churchill, London.

Ruffini, A. (1898). On the minute anatomy of the neuromuscular spindles of the cat and on their physiological significance. J. Physiol. (London) *23*, 190–208.

Starck, D. (1955). Embryologie. Thieme, Stuttgart.

Straus, W. L., and Rawles, M. E. (1953). An experimental study of the origin of the trunk musculature and ribs in the chick. Amer. J. Anat. *92*, 471–509.

Szent-Györgyi, A. (1948). The Nature of Life. A Study on Muscle. Academic Press, New York.

Szent-Györgyi, A. (1950). The Chemistry of Muscular Contraction 2nd ed. Academic Press, New York.

Szent-Györgyi, A. (1953). Chemical Physiology of Contraction in Body and Heart Muscle. Academic Press, New York.

Walls, E. W. (1960). The microanatomy of muscle. Chapter 2 *in* The Structure and Function of Muscle, Vol. I. G. H. Bourne (Ed.). Academic Press, New York & London.

Weinstock, I. M., and Iodice, A. A. (1969). Acid hydrolases in muscle wasting. Chapter 17 *in* Lysosomes in Biology and Pathology, Vol. I. J. T. Dingle and H. B. Fell (Eds.). North Holland Publishing Co., Amsterdam & London.

Willis, R. A. (1962). The Borderland of Embryology and Pathology. 2nd ed. Butterworths, London.

Yaffe, D., and Feldman, M. (1965). The formation of hybrid multinucleated muscle fibres from myoblasts of different genetic origin. Develop. Biol. *11*, 300–317.

Zacks, S. I. (1964). The Motor Endplate. W. B. Saunders Company, Philadelphia & London.

Chapter Two

Standard Reactions of Muscle

The anatomical and physiological characteristics of skeletal muscle determine its reaction to various altered states in its environment, and when we describe the pathological changes of muscle diseases we are constantly referring to either its altered physiology or to the morphological changes in the muscle fibres. Early experience of these changes came from observations on human diseases, but this knowledge has been expanded by creating certain pathological conditions of muscle in animal experiments. The account that follows, while including observations from human pathology, is primarily a summary of this experimental work.

DENERVATION

The consequences of the denervation of skeletal muscle have received more attention in human pathology and in animal experiments than any other aspect of muscle function. The literature is so large that only the more important papers and some recent reviews will be cited.

Important papers are those of Langley and Kato (1915), Langley (1917), Langley and Hashimoto (1918), Tower (1932, 1935, 1939), Denny-Brown and Pennybacker (1938) and Solandt and Magladery (1940, 1942). Among recent reviews, the multiauthor compilation edited by Gutmann (1962) and the large monograph of Sunderland (1968) are recommended.

It is convenient to divide the subject into the physiological and morphological changes of denervation. Only denervation due to a lesion of the lower motor neurone will be described here.

Physiological Changes of Denervation

The clinical signs of denervation of striated muscle are paresis or paralysis, hypotonia or flaccidity, diminished or absent tendon reflexes,

33

and fasciculation. To these signs may be added the information derived from the electrical stimulation and electrical recording of muscle. The important phenomenon of fibrillation is barely detectable as a physical sign in human disease.

PARALYSIS OR PARESIS

Paralysis of muscle is the sequel to the division of the motor (efferent) fibres which form the axons of the lower motor neurone. The lesion may be located in the spinal cord, the anterior spinal nerve roots, the peripheral nerve trunks, or the motor nerve endings. In the disease myasthenia gravis and also when certain paralysing drugs are used, there is physiological block between the motor end-plate and the muscle fibre.

HYPOTONIA

It is characteristic of a lower motor neurone denervation of muscle that the paralysis or paresis is *flaccid*. By this term we imply the loss of the normal reflex tone of innervated voluntary muscle. Hypotonia can also arise from sensory denervation of muscle as well as from lesions and degenerations of the cerebellum.

TENDON AREFLEXIA

Tendon reflexes are always either diminished or absent in lower motor neurone denervation, although this phenomenon may be masked by an accompanying lesion of the upper motor neurones. An excellent example of this coincidence of denervation caused by an upper and a lower motor neurone pathology is motor neurone disease, in which brisk tendon reflexes persist even in the later stages of the disease, when profound denervation atrophy is present in the muscles.

FASCICULATION

Fasciculation, unlike fibrillation, is a visible physical sign present in denervating human diseases, and is caused by the rapid spontaneous contraction of all the muscle fibres of a motor unit. The contraction of the group of muscles produces a small twitch, which is clearly seen through the skin during careful observation of the affected muscles. The term "fasciculation" was chosen by Denny-Brown and Pennybacker (1938) to distinguish this phenomenon from fibrillation.

Fasciculation is thought to be caused by a state of enhanced excitability of a motor unit which is sufficiently preserved to function in this uncoordinated manner. Fasciculation can result from a structural lesion of the neurone, apparently at any part of the perikaryon or its processes. It can also occur in and must be distinguished from certain causes of general neuronal excitability, such as electrolyte imbalance and the benign self-limiting condition of myokymia. Fasciculation is an important clinical sign in motor neurone disease and is also present in many other denervating diseases.

FIBRILLATION

Fibrillation is an abnormal contractile activity of denervated skeletal muscle. It is seen (best during operation exposure of the muscle) as fine rhythmical contractions, at intervals of 2 to 10 seconds, which cause a visible undulating movement of the surface of the muscle. Single muscle fibres or small groups of muscle fibres are affected; it is in this way that the phenomenon differs from fasciculation, in which the group of affected muscle fibres is larger and the activity may be detected through the skin as a clinical sign in human disease.

In man, fibrillation develops from 10 to 20 days after denervation, but the time interval depends on the muscle concerned and also on the distance of the nerve lesion from the spinal cord. The onset of fibrillation is more rapid when the nerve injury is near the muscle. Fibrillation persists for several years; probably as long as contractile protein survives in the muscle fibre.

The phenomenon of fibrillation has attracted much attention from research workers. It appears to be a fundamental property of the muscle cell, being seen in the isolated muscle cells grown in tissue cultures. In the normal adult muscle, fibrillation is restrained by the innervation of the muscle; consequently it appears when the innervation is lost. The appearance of fibrillation in denervated muscle coincides with important pharmacological changes, notably an enhanced sensitivity to the action of acetylcholine. Acetylcholine administered in small amounts to intact muscle will cause muscle activity similar to fibrillation. Fibrillation is of great interest in understanding the function of the muscle fibre, and its detection by electromyography is important in the investigation of patients. For the reasons stated, it cannot be observed as a clinical sign of denervation.

ELECTRICAL STIMULATION OF MUSCLE

Human or animal muscle may be stimulated electrically, either directly, by cutaneous electrodes placed over the surface of the muscle, or indirectly, by the stimulation of the nerve trunk supplying the muscle.

The electrical stimulus may be a continuous current (Galvanic stimulation) or a group of short pulses of current (Faradic stimulation). The altered excitability of denervated muscle to electrical stimulation was originally investigated by Erb (1868), and an excellent review is that of Licht (1961). The technique of investigating the electrical reaction of muscle is important because muscle fibres can be stimulated either directly or by stimulation of their nerve supply, either outside or within the muscle. The place at which the nerve enters the muscle (the motor point) is the area most responsive to electrical stimulation. Normal muscle responds to Galvanic and Faradic stimulation by a short duration contraction. With Galvanic stimulation the cathode-closing current produces a larger contraction than does the anode-closing current; this difference becomes greater as the strength of the electric current is increased. Denervated muscle gradually loses its electrical excitability, requiring stronger electrical currents and currents of longer duration to produce a contraction. The response to Faradic stimulation becomes feeble, and eventually cannot be elicited unless electrodes are inserted directly into the muscle. Galvanic stimulation continues to activate denervated muscle (as long as contractile protein remains), but the contraction is sluggish and prolonged. This combination of response to electrical stimulation — namely, loss of response to Faradic stimulation and the prolonged feeble response to Galvanic stimulation — is called the *reaction of degeneration.* Denervated muscle also responds differently in that the entire surface of the muscle is excitable and the contraction which occurs following stimulation is of the fibres in the neighbourhood of the stimulating electrode.

ELECTRICAL RECORDING OF MUSCLE

The use of electromyography in the diagnosis of human disease will be described in Chapter 10. Electrodes inserted into normal muscle at rest do not detect electrical activity after the stimulation of inserting the electrode has subsided. The electromyogram of denervated muscle records spontaneous action potentials that are the electrical counterpart of the visible fibrillation of individual muscle fibres and similarly persist as long as contractile protein is present in the muscle fibre. These characteristic potentials are sometimes called fibrillation potentials. They appear as monophasic or diphasic spikes of low amplitude, ranging from 5 to 100 microvolts, a short duration of 0.5 to 2 milliseconds, and a frequency of 2 to 20 per second (Sunderland, 1968).

Morphological Changes in Denervation

Following denervation, voluntary muscle undergoes a sequence of morphological changes which will be described under the following headings: *macroscopical appearances, microscopical appearances,* and *ultrastructural changes.*

MACROSCOPICAL APPEARANCES

The macroscopical appearances are chiefly those of atrophy, to which in the later stages may be added the features of *fibrosis* and *contrac-*

tures. The *atrophy* of voluntary muscle following denervation has been the subject of many studies, on a variety of experimental animals. Following experimental denervation, the appropriate muscle or muscles have been excised and weighed, and with groups of animals sacrificed at intervals, curves of the rates of denervation atrophy have been plotted (Sunderland, 1968). The nature of the curves obtained has been similar in the various experiments, and the following general conclusions may be stated. There is marked loss of weight within the first two months of denervation, following which the curve flattens. When the experiments have been prolonged, as by Gutmann (1948) for eight months in the rabbit and by Sunderland and Roy (1950) for 485 days in the oppossum, the weight loss after the third month has been very small. The percentage weight atrophy has varied up to 72 per cent and has always been greater than 50 per cent. *Fibrosis and contracture* has not been a feature of the experimental studies but is regularly seen clinically in human cases of muscle denervation. It is thought that fibrous contractures in human cases are caused by circulatory disturbances arising within the denervated muscle. These contractures must be distinguished from Volkmann's ischaemic contracture, in which there is a gross arterial pathology located outside the muscle but affecting a major artery supplying the muscle.

MICROSCOPICAL APPEARANCES

The microscopical appearance of denervated muscle has been extensively studied, both in experimental animals and in human cases (Fig. 2–1). The most important feature is the atrophy of the muscle fibre, which at 60 days after denervation may have its cross-sectional area reduced by 70 per cent (Fig. 2–2). In human cases the appearances depend on whether there is a single episode of rapid denervation (as in anterior poliomyelitis) or whether there is a chronic denervation (as in motor neurone disease) which may be complicated by reinnervation.

Bowden and Gutmann (1944) have made an extensive study of the microscopical appearances in muscle excised from human cases of denervation due to nerve injury. In the first three months they found atrophy of the muscle fibres, which increased towards the end of this period and which by the fourth month was considerable. The sarcolemmal nuclei were more numerous and were often arranged in rows or gathered in clumps. Central nuclei were sometimes seen. The intramuscular vessels were abnormal in that the tunica media of the arteries was thickened, with narrowing of the lumen. The intramuscular veins were dilated, with stasis of red cells. Several years after denervation the shrinkage of the muscle fibres had proceeded further, and connective tissue and fatty infiltration was present to a variable extent (Fig. 2–3). After periods of denervation of as long as 30 years the muscle was largely replaced by connective tissue and fat (Fig. 2–3).

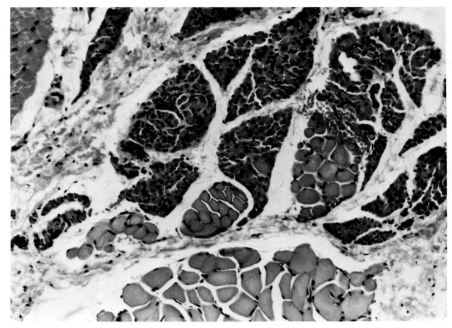

Figure 2–1 Group muscle fibre atrophy. Photomicrograph of a transverse section of the right triceps muscle from a 12-month-old girl suffering from Werdnig-Hoffmann disease. There are groups of atrophied muscle fibres adjacent to groups of muscle fibres of normal size. This is the typical histological picture of muscle undergoing chronic denervation. (Haematoxylin and eosin, × 210.)

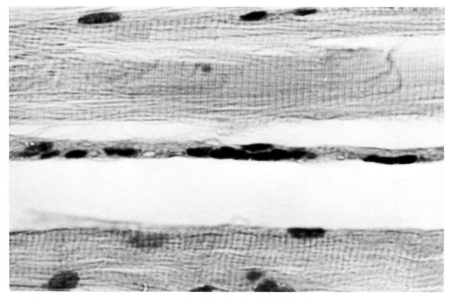

Figure 2–2 Extreme atrophy of a single muscle fibre. Photomicrograph of a longitudinal section from the quadriceps muscle of a case of peroneal muscular atrophy. The muscle fibre in the middle of the picture has atrophied to the point where only a group of sarcolemmal nuclei remain within the sarcolemmal sheath. (Haematoxylin and eosin, × 450.)

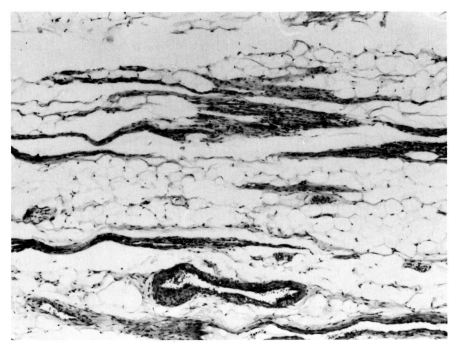

Figure 2–3 Fibrous and fatty replacement of denervated muscle. Photomicrograph of longitudinal section of quadriceps muscle from a case of acute poliomyelitis 15 years after the acute illness. The muscle has been largely replaced by connective tissue and fat. The remaining muscle fibres show severe denervation atrophy. (Haematoxylin and eosin, × 25.)

The effect of denervation on the intramuscular nerves and the motor end-plates probably depends on the efficiency of reinnervation. With severe or total denervation the axons within the muscle undergo wallerian degeneration, in which the myelin also is broken down (Bowden and Gutmann, 1944). The tubes of Schwann cell persist, providing evidence of denervation of the muscle. The motor end-plates were found by Tower (1935, 1939) to atrophy and disappear in six months, but other workers (reviewed by Sunderland, 1968) have found them to persist. Possibly the completeness of the denervation and the occurrence of reinnervation explains the discrepancies in the published accounts.

The effect of denervation on the muscle spindle requires special consideration. This was investigated experimentally by Tower (1932), who studied in cats the effect on the muscle spindles of sectioning separately the peripheral nerve, the anterior root, and the posterior root, and excising the sympathetic ganglia. Tower found that with peripheral nerve lesions the muscle spindles atrophied to the same extent as did the other (extrafusal) muscle fibres. The final result was the replacement of the atrophied muscle spindle with fibrous tissue and an increase of the capsular connective tissue. Anterior root section produced atrophy of the polar part of the spindle, while posterior root section caused atrophy of the equatorial region. Sympathetic denervation had no effect.

In human denervating diseases and in human muscle denervated by peripheral nerve injuries, the changes are probably similar to those found experimentally. In the peripheral neuropathy of peroneal muscular atrophy, atrophy and fibrosis of the muscle spindles is a constant finding (Hughes and Brownell, 1972), while in the denervating diseases located primarily in the spinal cord the muscle spindles are usually conspicuously preserved.

ULTRASTRUCTURE OF DENERVATED MUSCLE

The ultrastructural changes in denervated voluntary muscle have been studied experimentally (Wechsler and Hager, 1961; Pellegrino and Franzini, 1963; Lee and Altschul, 1963), and by muscle biopsy in human denervating diseases. Roth, Graziani, Terry and Scheinberg (1965) described the appearances in the Kugelberg-Welander syndrome; Afifi, Aleu, Goodgold and MacKay (1966) those in amyotrophic lateral sclerosis; and Hughes and Brownell (1969) those in Werdnig-Hoffmann disease. From these studies has been constructed a reasonably complete picture of the ultrastructural changes of the muscle fibre undergoing denervation (Figs. 2–4 to 2–10).

The atrophy of the muscle fibre is again conspicuous, and in muscle from Werdnig-Hoffmann disease, muscle fibres with a diameter of 4 μm were observed representing a ten- to twentyfold diminution of the muscle fibre size (Fig. 2–4). The sarcolemmal nuclei show changes. There is a moderate contraction in size that is mainly evident as a complex infolding of the nuclear membrane, as distinct from the simple folds seen in the nuclei of normal muscle fibres.

The *band structure* of the muscle fibre is disorganised (Fig. 2–5). The earliest change is a lack of distinction of the A, I and Z bands. This blurring of the band structure is due to two phenomena. The first is a loss of alignment of the bands across neighbouring myofibrils; this is slight at first, but later, when whole myofibrils are lost, the band structure becomes very uneven. The second cause of the indistinct band structure is loss of myofilaments; this loss is proportionate to the atrophy of the muscle fibre. This disorder of the band structure is a very sensitive index of denervation, and ranges from a slight unevenness of the bands to complete disorganisation, with no ordered orientation of the few surviving myofilaments (Fig. 2–6). The *myofibrils* become smaller in the early stages as the result of a progressive loss of myofilaments. At a later stage, some myofibrils appear to be broken up, and finally no myofibrillar arrangement can be recognised at all (Fig. 2–7). The number of

(*Text continued on page 44.*)

Figures **2–4** to **2–10** are electron micrographs showing the ultrastructure of denervated muscle from a case of Werdnig-Hoffmann disease. (Case 1 described in Hughes and Brownell, 1968.)

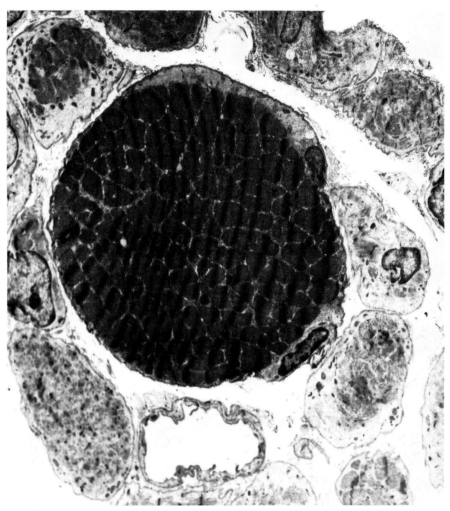

Figure 2–4 Group of denervated muscle fibres seen in transverse section. The large round central muscle fibre is normal. The small size of the surrounding denervated muscle fibres can be judged by comparison with the size of the capillary at the bottom of the picture. (Phosphotungstic acid, × 6000.)

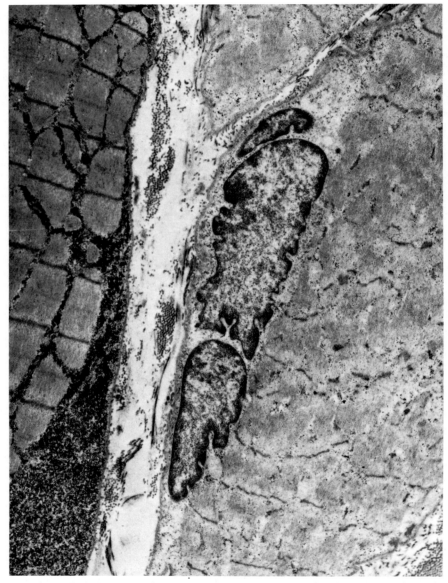

Figure 2–5 Denervated muscle fibre (*right*) compared with adjacent normal muscle fibre (*left*). Note the blurring of the band structure in the denervated muscle fibre. (2% aqueous uranyl acetate/lead citrate, × 8000.)

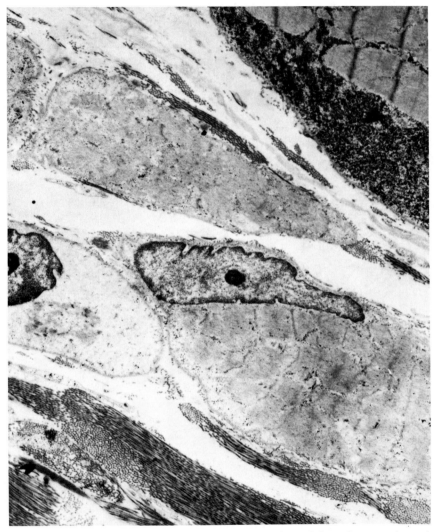

Figure 2–6 Detail of a normal muscle fibre (*top right*) and three denervated muscle fibres showing differing stages of denervation. One fibre (*bottom right*) shows early denervation with blurring of the band structure. Another fibre (*top left*) shows more advanced denervation and one fibre (*middle left*) shows complete loss of contractile material except for a single surviving myofibril. (2% aqueous uranyl acetate/lead citrate, × 8000.)

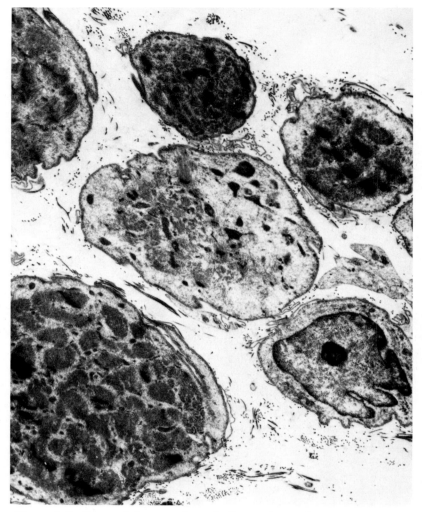

Figure 2–7 Group of denervated muscle fibres. The band structure is grossly disorganised but surviving portions of the Z bands can be identified. The myofilaments are disorientated and some which are seen in longitudinal section are adjacent to others seen in transverse section. Note the redundant folds of the sarcolemma. (Phosphotungstic acid, × 8000.)

myofilaments progressively diminishes; the peripheral region of the muscle fibre being the area first depleted (Fig. 2–8). The number of *mitochondria* in denervated muscle fibres varies; sometimes excessive numbers are present.

The *sarcolemma* shows an interesting change. The double layer of the sarcolemmal sheath is preserved even in the most atrophied muscle

(*Text continued on page 49.*)

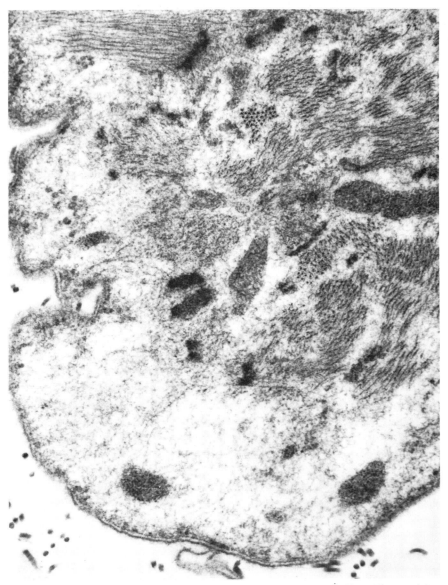

Figure 2–8 Detail of transverse sections of denervated muscle fibre. The surviving myofilaments have lost any orderly alignment. Some are seen in transverse section adjacent to others cut longitudinally. (Phosphotungstic acid, × 8000.)

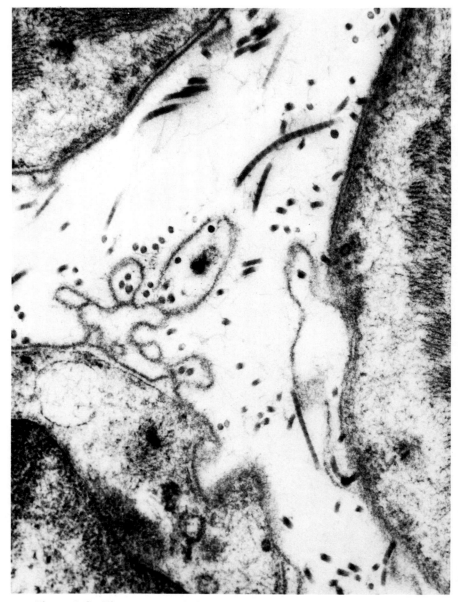

Figure 2–9 Ultrastructure of the sarcolemma of denervated muscle fibres. The double layer of the sarcolemmal sheath can be seen. The inner layer (the cytolemma) still invests closely the atrophied muscle fibre but the outer layer (the basement membrane) appears as redundant folds. (Phosphotungstic acid, × 33,000.)

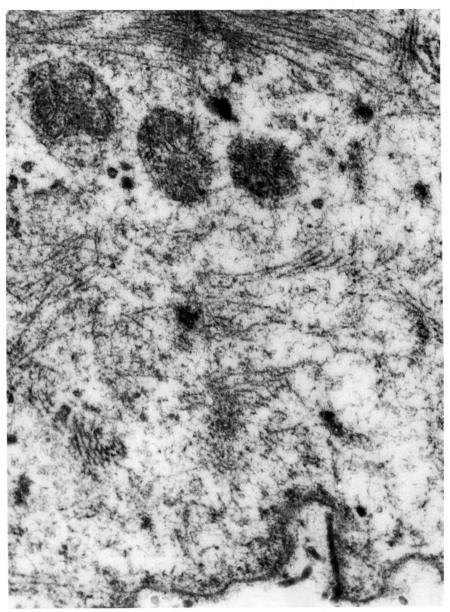

Figure 2-10 Peripheral (subsarcolemmal) part of muscle fibre undergoing early denervation. Note the loss of myofilaments from the subsarcolemmal region where only a few myofilaments, orientated in several directions, can be seen. (Phosphotungstic acid, × 40,000.)

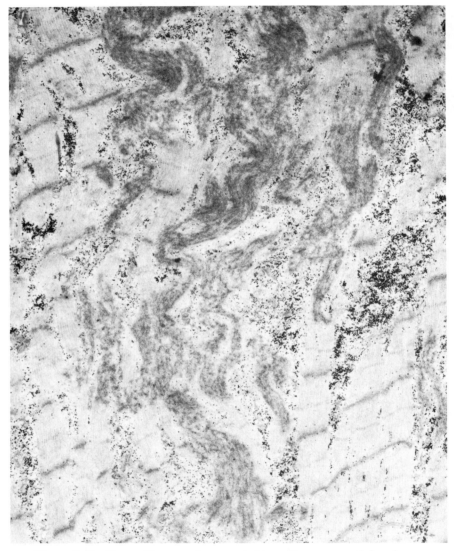

Figure 2–11   Target fibre seen in a muscle biopsy from a case of chronic neuropathy. The electron micrograph shows the centre of a target fibre cut in longitudinal section. The central area contains a core of electron-dense material similar to that making up the normal Z-line (2% aqueous uranyl acetate/lead citrate, × 15,000.)

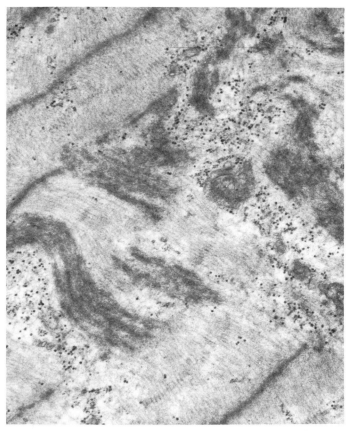

Figure 2–12 Target fibre. Higher magnification of electron-dense material. (2% aqueous uranyl acetate/lead citrate, × 26,500.)

fibres, and the sarcolemmal sheath is folded to accommodate the reduction in size of the muscle fibre. The inner layer (the cytolemma) still invests closely the atrophied muscle fibre, but the outer layer (the basement membrane) gives off large redundant folds, often of considerable size (Fig. 2–9). The *sarcoplasmic reticulum* initially shows enlargement, but later, when the muscle fibre is disorganised, few elements of this reticulum or of the tubular system can be recognised.

In muscle fibres undergoing denervation there sometimes appears a central column of structural change, involving several adjacent myofibrils which are replaced by electron-dense material resembling that which normally makes up the Z line (Figs. 2–11 and 2–12). From the light microscopical appearance of these muscle fibres, as seen in transverse section, they have been named target fibres (Engel, 1961). They are now known to occur also in disorders not obviously associated with denervation.

TRAUMA

The reaction of the mammalian striated muscle to trauma has been the subject of many experimental studies using different animals and varying the manner in which the trauma is applied. Experiments have been performed with cutting, crushing, and the application of heat and of cold (Adams, Denny-Brown and Pearson, 1962). An excellent account of an experimental study is that of Clark (1946) and of Clark and Wajda (1947). The nature of the experimental lesion depends partly on the method of causing the trauma, but a more important distinction is whether the muscle fibre is only partially damaged or whether it is completely destroyed by the trauma.

An example of partial damage to the fibre is a clean transverse cut across a muscle. This incision into the muscle is rapidly filled with blood clot and exuded protein fluid. The two cut ends of the muscle fibre appear as partially emptied sarcolemmal tubes, the contents of which retract from the area of the cut and leave the tubes empty for a distance of a few millimetres. Within one or two days the area of the cut has an exudate of polymorphs and monocytes with new capillaries and fibroblasts. At the same time, the sarcolemmal nuclei of the injured muscle fibres become rounded, and by the third day some of the tissue histiocytes have

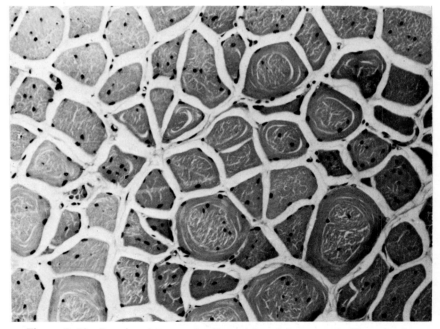

Figure 2–13 Regenerating muscle fibres injured by trauma. Note the intense nuclear activity and the ring fibres. (Haematoxylin and eosin, × 210.)

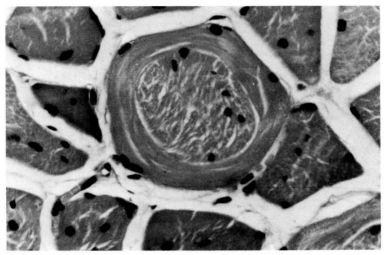

Figure 2–14   Ring fibre. A thin layer of myofibrils at the periphery of the muscle fibre encircles the normally directed central body of myofibrils. (Haematoxylin and eosin, ×400.)

entered the sarcolemmal tubes. The sarcolemmal nuclei now appear very active and possibly there is nuclear division, although actual mitoses have not been seen (Figs. 2–13 to 2–15). After one week the cut end of the sarcolemmal tube forms a growth bud which, if the intervening dis-

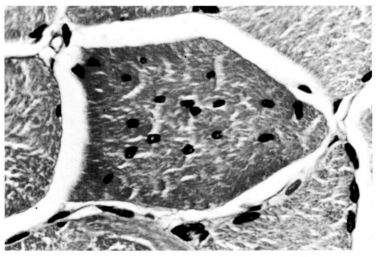

Figure 2–15   Muscle fibre regenerating after trauma. Note the numerous central sarcolemmal nuclei. (Haematoxylin and eosin, ×550.)

tance is short, fuses with a bud from a muscle fibre on the other side of the cut. These buds consist of regenerated sarcoplasm with many sarcolemmal nuclei (Figs. 2–16 and 2–17). In time, these multicellular buds fuse and the signs of reparative activity subside. Within one month the anatomy of the muscle fibre is largely restored.

The histological appearance of the muscle following a crushing injury or following coagulation from heat or cold is complex. This is because some of the muscle fibres are so badly damaged that they are removed and replaced by connective tissue, resulting in the formation of a connective tissue scar within the muscle. Nevertheless, there is considerable regeneration of partially damaged muscle fibres, and large numbers of developing muscle buds can be found in the second and third week after this type of trauma. The application of heat and cold produces the phenomenon of "shredded" necrosis, which consists of irregular transverse striations, probably caused by the violent contraction of the muscle fibre induced by the stimulus.

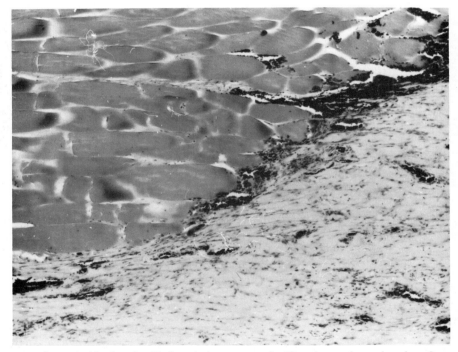

Figure 2–16 Repair of infarct in human muscle. The picture shows the edge of an infarct in muscle caused by embolism. Above and to the left is undamaged muscle. To the right and below is granulation tissue which is being replaced by growing muscle fibres. (Haematoxylin and eosin, × 95.)

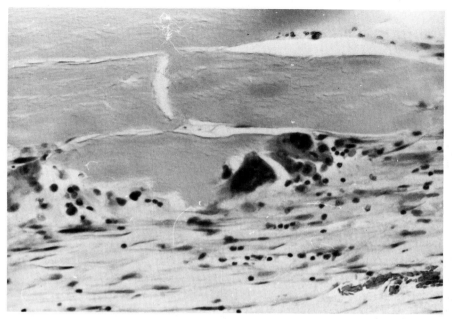

Figure 2–17 Detail of regenerating muscle seen in the area between the infarcted muscle and normal muscle in Figure 2–16. Note the sprouting buds of muscle fibres. (Haematoxylin and eosin, × 240.)

ISCHAEMIA

The subject of muscle ischaemia is of considerable importance in both accident and orthopaedic surgery, and there will be a more extensive discussion of this subject in Chapter 9. Here, only a summary of experimental work will be given. Several thorough experimental studies have been made and the following accounts are recommended: Brooks, 1922; Clark, 1946; Harman, 1947; and Harman and Gwinn, 1949.

The experimental work has been done mainly on rabbits and rats. The acute ischaemia has been produced by the ligation of several nutrient muscle arteries passing to an individual muscle, by the application of tourniquets to limbs, or by the temporary excision and replacement of a muscle. This variety of experimental procedures has allowed a range in the severity of the ischaemia, the most severe being produced by the method last described. Clark, in some of his experiments, excised and replaced a rectangular portion about 15 mm long of the gracilis muscle in rabbits. At three days the graft had the appearance of a yellow slough, which was unstained by bromophenol blue injected into the animal 10 minutes before the animal was killed. Microscopy of the grafted muscle showed it to be composed of dead muscle fibres devoid of nuclei and undergoing fragmentation. The connective tissue of the endomysium was also largely destroyed, apart from an occasional fibrocyte. At the margins of the grafts, some muscle fibres or portions of muscle fibres were still preserved, presumably because of the proximity of the vessels in the adjacent tissues. These surviving muscle fibres showed basophilia and, with fat stains, an increase of fat granules could be demonstrated.

At one week, the appearance in the centre of the graft was the same, but on the outside, sprouting plasmodial buds were growing into the graft from the neighbouring muscle, and there was similar regeneration activity in the peripheral margin of the muscle graft. At 11 days, by bromophenol blue injection, the graft was shown to have a blood supply and was now invaded by young fibroblastic tissue in which layers of parallel regenerated muscle fibres could be recognised. These fibres were about half the diameter of normal muscle fibres and already the cross striations could be detected. They arose mostly by inward growth from the surrounding muscle, but also partly from surviving muscle fibres within the graft (Figs. 2–16 and 2–17). From several published accounts it is clear that within three or four weeks after ischaemic infarction the damaged muscle is largely replaced.

DISUSE ATROPHY

Voluntary muscle possesses the properties of hypertrophy in response to excessive exercise and atrophy in response to disuse. The phenomenon of disuse atrophy is well known in medical practice, both in disabling diseases and following immobilisation procedures, particularly the treatment of fractures. Only when the innervation of the muscles concerned is intact can we describe the atrophy as disuse atrophy.

In animal experiments, disuse atrophy has been produced by isolating several segments of the spinal cord by transections above and below; by detaching the muscle from its principal insertion by a tenotomy operation; and by immobilising limbs by splinting or encasement in plaster casts. All of these methods will produce disuse atrophy, but there are many technical difficulties in ensuring that the muscle is at rest. In successful experiments there is a progressive shrinkage in volume and loss of weight of the appropriate muscles. The amount of muscle atrophy produced varies with the species used, the muscles chosen and the techniques applied. Sunderland (1968) has reviewed the reports of these experiments; in which a weight loss of up to 50 per cent is common. This *disuse atrophy* in animal experiments is less conspicuous than denervation atrophy. One interesting feature that has emerged from histochemical studies is that disuse atrophy, as produced by tenotomy experiments (Engel, Brooke and Nelson, 1966), affects the granular (type I) fibres much more than the agranular (type II) fibres.

Sunderland and Lavarack (1959) have reported studies on human cases of tenotomy and amputation, and have described in detail the appearances of the muscles in human disuse atrophy. The muscles rendered inactive were paler than normal, but retained their general form and texture. Even after many years they were still recognisable as muscles, and did not merge into surrounding connective tissue. The muscles showed a marked reduction in size and weight: usually more than a 50 per cent and sometimes more than a 60 per cent weight loss. Microscopically the muscle fibres were atrophied, sometimes to an extreme degree. The numbers and form of the sarcolemmal nuclei appeared normal and the striations of the muscle fibres were usually preserved. Some muscle fibres showed severe degenerative changes, with vacuolar fragmentation of the sarcoplasm and a round cell reaction. The motor end-plates and the muscle spindles were not observed to be abnormal. The connective tissue throughout the atrophied muscle appeared increased both in the fibrous sheath of the endomysium and in the perimysium, but calculations showed that this was probably a condensation of the normal quantity of connective tissue into the smaller volume of the atrophied muscle belly. In fact these authors thought that, when one considered absolute quantities, there was a moderate diminution of connective tissue in the muscles of disuse atrophy. The vessels were not observed to be abnormal.

References

Adams, R. D., Denny-Brown, D., and Pearson, C. M. (1962). Diseases of Muscle. A Study in Pathology. 2nd ed. Harper & Row, New York.

Afifi, A. K., Aleu, F. P., Goodgold, J., and Mackay, B. (1966). Ultrastructure of atrophic muscle in amyotrophic lateral sclerosis. Neurology (Minneap.) *16*, 475–481.

Bowden, R. E. M., and Gutmann, E. (1944). Denervation and reinnervation of human voluntary muscle. Brain *67*, 273–313.

Brooks, B. (1922). Pathologic changes in muscle as a result of disturbances of circulation: An experimental study of Volkmann's ischemic paralysis. Arch. Surg. *5*, 18–216.

Clark, W. E. LeG. (1946). An experimental study of the regeneration of mammalian striped muscle. J. Anat. *80*, 24–36.

Clark, W. E. LeG., and Wajda, H. S. (1947). The growth and maturation of regenerating striated muscle fibres. J. Anat. *81*, 56–63.

Denny-Brown, D., and Pennybacker, J. B. (1938). Fibrillation and fasciculation in voluntary muscle. Brain *61*, 311–334.

Engel, W. K. (1961). Muscle target fibres, a newly recognized sign of denervation. Nature (London) *191*, 389–390.

Engel, W. K., Brooke, M. H., and Nelson, P. G. (1966). Histochemical studies of denervated or tenotomized cat muscle: illustrating difficulties in relating experimental animal conditions to human neuromuscular disorders. Ann. N.Y. Acad. Sci. *138*, 160–185.

Erb, W. (1868). Zur Pathologie und pathologischen Anatomie peripherischen Paralysen. Dtsch. Arch. klin. Med. *4*, 534–578.

Gutmann, E. (1948). Effect of delay of innervation on recovery of muscle after nerve lesions. J. Neurophysiol. *11*, 279–294.

Gutmann, E. (1962). The Denervated Muscle. Academia, Czechoslovak Academy of Sciences, Prague.

Harman, J. W. (1947). A histologic study of skeletal muscle in acute ischaemia. Amer. J. Path. *23*, 551–566.

Harman, J. W., and Gwinn, R. P. (1949). The recovery of skeletal muscle fibres from acute ischaemia, as determined by histological and chemical methods. Amer. J. Path. 25, 741–, 756.

Hughes, J. T., and Brownell, B. (1972). Pathology of peroneal muscular atrophy (Charcot-Marie-Tooth disease). J. Neurol. Neurosurg. Psychiat. 35, 648–657.

Hughes, J. T., and Brownell, B. (1969). Ultrastructure of muscle in Werdnig-Hoffman Disease. J. Neurol. Sci. 8, 363–379.

Langley, J. N. (1917). Observations on denervated and on regenerating muscle. J. Physiol. (London) 51, 377–395.

Langley, J. N., and Hashimoto, M. (1918). Observations on the atrophy of denervated muscle. J. Physiol. (London) 52, 15–69.

Langley, J. N., and Kato, T. (1915). The rate of loss of weight in skeletal muscle after nerve section with some observations on the effect of stimulation and other treatment. J. Physiol. (London) 49, 432–440.

Lee, J. C., and Altschul, R. (1963). Electron microscopy of the nuclei of denervated skeletal muscle. Z. Zellforsch. 61, 168–182.

Licht, S. (1961). Electrodiagnosis and Electromyography. 2nd ed. New Haven, Connecticut. Published by the author.

Pellegrino, C., and Franzini, C. (1963). An electron microscope study of denervation atrophy in red and white skeletal muscle fibres. J. Cell. Biol. 17, 327–349.

Roth, R. G., Graziani, L. J., Terry, R. D., and Scheinberg, L. C. (1965). Muscle fibre structure in the Kugelberg-Welander syndrome (chronic spinal muscular atrophy). J. Neuropath. Exp. Neurol. 24, 444–454.

Solandt, D. Y., and Magladery, J. W. (1940). The relation of atrophy to fibrillation in denervated muscle. Brain 63, 255–263.

Solandt, D. Y., and Magladery, J. W. (1942). A comparison of effects of upper and lower motor neurone lesions of skeletal muscles. J. Neurophysiol. 5, 373–380.

Sunderland, S. (1968). Nerves and Nerve Injuries. Livingstone, Edinburgh & London.

Sunderland, S., and Lavarack, J. O. (1959). Changes in human muscles after permanent tenotomy. J. Neurol. Neurosurg. Psychiat. 22, 167–174.

Sunderland, S., and Roy, L. J. (1950). Denervation changes in mammalian striated muscle. J. Neurol. Neurosurg. Psychiat. 13, 159–177.

Tower, S. S. (1932). Atrophy and degeneration in the muscle spindle. Brain 55, 77–90.

Tower, S. S. (1935). Atrophy and degeneration in skeletal muscle. Amer. J. Anat. 56, 1–44.

Tower, S. S. (1939). Reaction of muscle to denervation. Physiol. Rev. 19, 1–48.

Wechsler, W., and Hager, H. (1961). Electronenmikroskopische Befunde bei Muskelatrophie nach Nervendurchtrennung bei der weissen Ratte. Beitr. path. Anat. 125, 31–53.

Chapter Three

Denervating Diseases

An important group of diseases causing muscle weakness or muscle atrophy are the denervating diseases, a miscellany of conditions whose common factor is the denervation of voluntary muscle. These diseases are important in their own right, but also must be studied in order that they may be distinguished from the primary muscle diseases.

Denervating diseases can be classified according to the anatomical situation of the lesion in the nervous system. The initial subdivision is to distinguish whether the paresis or paralysis is due to a disorder of the upper motor neurone, to the extrapyramidal part of the nervous system, or to a disorder of the lower motor neurone. While some remarks on the first type will be made later, it is with the last named group that we are chiefly concerned, and this group can be further subdivided. The lower motor neurone can be damaged by disease of either the neurone cell body, the spinal nerve roots, the peripheral nerve trunks, or the motor nerve endings and the neuromuscular apparatus. Details of only the most important of these diseases will be given, but some other causes of denervation will be listed. An excellent classification of the neuromuscular disorders has been compiled by Gardner-Medwin and Walton (1969).

This division into four anatomical sites of disease is useful and, for most of the conditions to be considered, appropriate; however, in some diseases, (e.g., motor neurone disease), the whole neurone is affected, and such diseases cannot be assigned with certainty to any one group.

DISORDERS OF THE NEURONE CELL BODY

There are many examples of diseases causing damage to the peri-karyon of the neurone. The disease may be acute (anterior poliomyelitis) or chronic (syringomyelia). The following diseases in this category will be described: *anterior poliomyelitis, spinal cord trauma, syringomyelia, intrame-*

57

dullary tumours, anterior spinal artery occlusion, Werdnig-Hoffmann disease, and motor neurone disease.

Other diseases in this group, which will be listed but not discussed further, are herpes zoster; spinal cord transections due to extramedullary tumours, abscesses, etc.; neural tube malformations; Kugelberg-Welander disease; and variants of motor neurone disease associated with heredofamilial ataxias.

Anterior Poliomyelitis

Formerly this was a widespread endemic and epidemic disease mainly of white races in temperate climates and occurring naturally only in human populations. The successful introduction of an effective vaccine has dramatically reduced the incidence in developed countries. It remains a hazard of countries in which an effective vaccination programme has not been carried out. It is also important to note that denervation atrophy may be present from a mild attack of this disease several

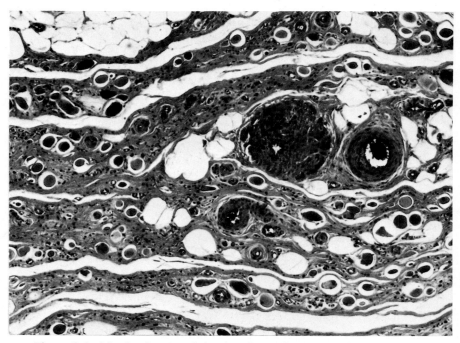

Figure 3–1 Muscle denervated by anterior poliomyelitis. Photomicrograph of transverse section of psoas muscle examined 12 years after the acute neurological disease. There are isolated muscle fibres seen among fibrous tissue and fat. Note the large but narrowed blood vessels supplying the inactive muscle. (Haematoxylin and eosin, × 105.)

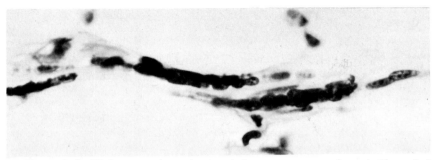

Figure 3–2 High power photomicrograph from same case as shown in Figure 3–1. Two severely atrophied muscle fibres are seen in longitudinal sections. The sarcolemmal nuclei are crowded together in the atrophied fibres which consist largely of sarcolemmal tubes. (Haematoxylin and eosin, × 500.)

years previously. Such a finding in a patient now presenting with another neuromuscular disease may cause diagnostic difficulty.

The findings in the skeletal muscles after an attack of acute anterior poliomyelitis depend on the extent and location of the acute disease and the time interval that has elapsed. In the acute stage of the disease there may be inflammatory changes in the muscle (Bowden, 1952), probably due to the acute denervation. For some time after the acute disease there may be the type of denervation changes that suggest a myopathy (Drachman, Murphy, Nigam and Hills, 1967). The late stages of denervation from poliomyelitis are familiar: the muscle shows an extreme degree of fatty and fibrous tissue replacement of the lost muscle fibres (Figs. 3–1 and 3–2).

Spinal Cord Trauma

In spinal injuries affecting the cervical and thoracic regions of the spinal cord, sensory loss and an upper motor neurone paralysis below the cord transection dominate the clinical picture. Lower motor neurone paralysis is always present, but is not usually clinically evident in the thoracic region of the cord. In damage to the lumbosacral part of the spinal cord, lower motor neurone paralysis may be prominent, particularly when the cauda equina is also involved. In these circumstances the muscles of the lower limbs frequently show conspicuous denervation atrophy.

Syringomyelia

Syringomyelia (Hughes, 1966) may be primary or secondary, the latter group being caused by either tumours or trauma. Primary syringomyelia must be distinguished from hydromyelia, which is a dilatation of the central canal of the spinal cord.

The syrinx in primary syringomyelia usually occupies the upper part of the spinal cord and may extend into the medulla. It is usually a central but may sometimes be an asymmetrical one-sided cavitation frequently involving the anterior horns of the cervical enlargement. Lower motor neurone denervation of the arm muscles may be present, and has to be distinguished clinically from motor neurone disease.

The muscles of the upper limbs, particularly the small muscles of the hand and the forearm muscles, may show severe denervation atrophy. The chronicity of this denervation will usually distinguish the histological appearances in the muscle from those found in motor neurone disease.

Intramedullary Tumours

Intramedullary tumours are mostly primary, but the rare secondary tumour will cause a similar syndrome of cord transection and lower motor neurone paralysis from destruction of the anterior horns. The diagnosis is usually apparent without examination of muscle being required.

Anterior Spinal Artery Occlusion

This condition characteristically causes extensive damage to the anterior grey horns. Either the upper part or the lower part of the artery is involved, usually as a secondary phenomenon caused by some other pathology affecting the artery (Hughes and Brownell, 1964). In the commoner "upper" type there is, in the acute stage, a cord transection with a severe effect on the cervical enlargement. If the patient survives the acute episode, the long tract changes may recover, leaving the patient with lower motor paralysis of several muscles in the upper limbs. This is the stage causing the important clinical syndrome of denervation atrophy.

Werdnig-Hoffmann Disease

This is a system degeneration of anterior horn motor neurones. It is inherited as an autosomal recessive condition. The main abnormalities are in the motor nuclei of the cranial nerves and in the anterior horns of the spinal cord. In the spinal cord the long tracts are normal but the anterior horns show loss of large motor neurones. Neuronophagia of affected neurone cell bodies can be seen.

The appearance of the skeletal muscles is very characteristic of the disease (Hughes and Brownell, 1969), and a muscle biopsy is a valuable aid to diagnosis. The muscle fibres show atrophy of large connected groups, the distribution being that of the "group atrophy" reminiscent of motor neurone disease. Between the groups of atrophied muscle fibres are groups of mainly normal muscle fibres but often with an occasional atrophied fibre. The muscle spindles are normal and are often prominent among the other atrophied muscle fibres. The small intramuscular nerve endings show fibre loss.

Motor Neurone Disease

Under this name are included three conditions formerly considered as independent diseases—progressive muscular atrophy, amyotrophic lateral sclerosis, and progressive bulbar paralysis (Hughes, 1966). The component of this disease which concerns us here is the progressive

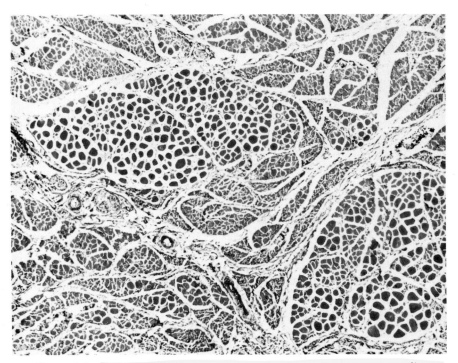

Figure 3-3 Group muscle fibre atrophy seen in a case of motor neurone disease. The picture is from a histological section of biceps brachii examined at necropsy. Note the two bundles of normal muscle fibres (*upper left* and *lower right*) which stand out by comparison with the other atrophied muscle fibres. (Haematoxylin and eosin, ×60.)

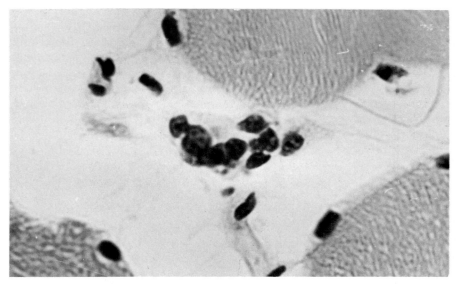

Figure 3-4 Chronic denervation seen in a case of peroneal muscular atrophy at necropsy. The picture is from a transverse section of the peroneal longus. Between two normal muscle fibres is a grossly atrophied muscle fibre seen in transverse section. The group of sarcolemmal nuclei must not be mistaken for inflammatory cells. (Haematoxylin and eosin, × 500.)

lower motor neurone paralysis of the limbs and of the muscles supplied by the cranial nerves.

The skeletal muscles in this condition always show important changes that can frequently be used to diagnose the condition. For biopsy, arm or leg muscles may be examined; probably a portion of the deltoid muscle or of the vastus lateralis muscle is most convenient. At necropsy the intrinsic muscles of the hands and feet give good opportunities for examining the nerve supply of the muscles in this disease. The histological appearance of the muscle is very characteristic (Fig. 3–3). In transverse or longitudinal section we find groups of atrophied muscle fibres among fibres of normal size. Sometimes only one or two atrophied fibres can be seen in one area, but more commonly a whole fasciculus composed of atrophied muscle fibres is found. This is the group atrophy characteristic of this disease.

DISORDERS OF THE SPINAL NERVE ROOTS

Only a few of the many different causes of lesions of spinal nerve roots will be mentioned here. A more detailed description would be out of place because in most of these conditions the denervation of muscle is only incidental to the disease. It is, however, important to know of these causes of denervation, which in some instances (e.g., denervation seen in an upper limb muscle biopsy from a patient with cervical spondylosis) will cause difficulty in the interpretation of a muscle biopsy.

Diseases of the spine involving the intervertebral foraminae (e.g., spondylosis, osteoarthritis and Paget's disease) frequently compress spinal nerve roots. Other spinal diseases with osteoporosis may cause root compression indirectly, as the result of gross structural deformity of the spine.

Both benign and malignant tumours can affect nerve roots. Of the benign tumours, the meningioma and the neurofibroma are the most frequent causes of nerve root compression. Of malignant tumours, most cases of root compression are caused by secondary carcinomas and reticuloses.

The acute polyradiculopathy of Guillain-Barré disease consists of a widespread paralysis caused by extensive demyelination of the peripheral nerves. Some axonal degeneration is usually present in the condition, and the disease process is most intense in the region of the spinal nerve roots. In the acute disease it is unlikely that a muscle biopsy will be required for diagnosis. A biopsy in this acute phase would show very few changes, and probably these would be confined to degeneration of the terminal nerve endings in the muscle (Figs. 3–5 and 3–6). More

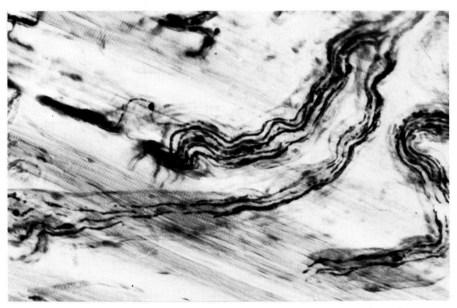

Figure 3–5 Landry's paralysis. Acute neuronal degeneration seen in an intramuscular nerve stained by a silver technique. (Schofield, × 180.)

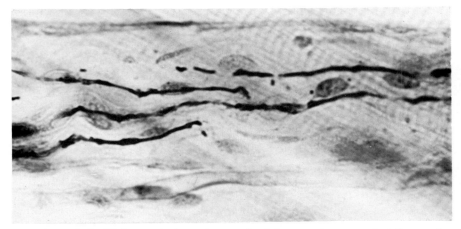

Figure 3–6 High power photomicrograph of degenerating nerve bundle seen in Figure 3–5. (Schofield, × 500.)

important, however, is that following recovery from the disease there may be residual axonal degeneration appearing in the muscles as denervation atrophy.

Toxic causes of damage to spinal nerve roots are mainly instances when toxic substances are injected intrathecally. Alcohol and solutions of phenol are injected intrathecally to relieve severe pain or intractable spasticity. These intrathecal procedures, which are usually employed in the lumbosacral region, act mainly by causing a toxic radiculitis, and are most effective when they injure the cauda equina. Occasionally, spinal anaesthetic solutions have a similar but unplanned effect.

DISORDERS OF THE PERIPHERAL NERVE TRUNKS

Trauma is the commonest cause of localised nerve lesions, which may result either from a single acute injury or from chronic recurrent trauma, as in the entrapment neuropathies.

There are many toxic causes of peripheral neuropathy but most of these are rare. The most important toxic agents are arsenic, lead, mercury, thallium, triorthocresylphosphate, isoniazide, nitrofurantoin, thalidomide and insulin. The neuropathies of uraemia and porphyria may also be toxic, but result from an endogenous toxin elaborated in the body. Nutritional causes of polyneuropathy are mainly varieties of vitamin B deficiency, which occurs in certain famine states (beri-beri, pellagra), in chronic alcoholism, and in cases of deficient diets due to mental disorders, senility, and chronic illnesses. The cause of the neuropathy associated with carcinomatosis and reticulosis is unknown and may prove to be either toxic or nutritional. The neuropathy found in myelomatosis may have a cause similar to that in other malignant condi-

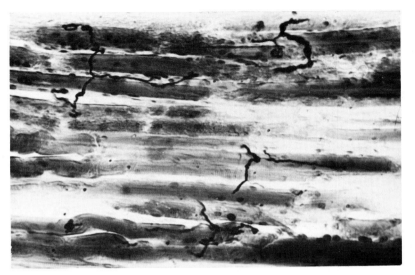

Figure 3-7   Chronic neuropathy. Extensor digitorum muscle (necropsy specimen) from a case of peroneal muscular atrophy. The terminations of the nerves show thickenings and other irregularities. (Schofield, × 120.)

tions, but sometimes is due to amyloid deposition in the nerves. Amyloidosis of peripheral nerves can occur in either primary or secondary amyloid states.

The polyneuropathy of Guillain-Barré disease has already been mentioned; a similar condition can follow the exanthematous diseases of childhood. An important group of neuropathies occur in the collagen

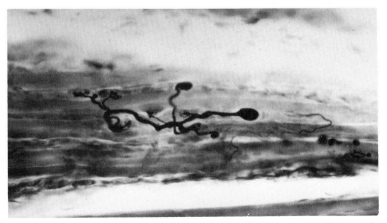

Figure 3-8   Chronic neuropathy. Thenar muscle from a case of peroneal muscular atrophy. There is branching and thickening of the terminal arborization with several growth cones. (Schofield, × 200.)

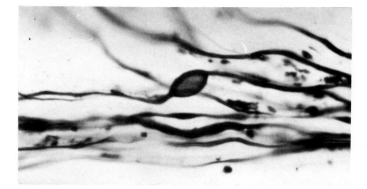

Figure 3–9 Chronic neuropathy. Vastus lateralis muscle from a case of peroneal muscular atrophy. The picture shows loss of axons and an axonic swelling. (Schofield, × 1400.)

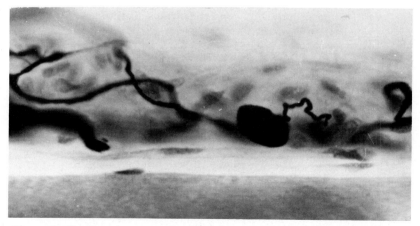

Figure 3–10 Chronic neuropathy. Growth cone at the end of a regenerating axon. (Schofield, × 1400.)

diseases, rheumatoid arthritis, polyarteritis nodosa, disseminated lupus erythematosus and systemic sclerosis; sarcoidosis may also be considered with this group. Inherited diseases with neuropathy include peroneal muscular atrophy (Figs. 3–7 to 3–10), hypertrophic interstitial neuropathy, and congenital sensory neuropathy. Leprosy is the only common bacterial disease involving nerve trunks, which in the neurocutaneous form of this disease are consistently attacked. It has been recently discovered that the leprosy bacillus invades the muscle fibre; this phenomenon will be described in Chapter 6.

DISORDERS OF THE MOTOR NERVE ENDINGS AND THE NEUROMUSCULAR APPARATUS

Axonal degeneration from whatever cause will result in degeneration of the terminal intramuscular nerves, and this phenomenon (often accompanied by signs of regeneration) may be expected in a wide variety of denervating conditions. In some diseases (e.g., motor neurone disease) and toxic states (e.g., triorthocresylphosphate toxicity), there is a tendency for the terminal part of the neurone to show more advanced changes than any other part. This feature is known as the "dying back" of the neurone, the supposition being that at its terminal extremity the nutrition of the axon is at its most precarious. This phenomenon of "dying back" of the neurone is best demonstrated in muscle in cases of Werdnig-Hoffmann disease. The motor axons characteristically continue to the last millimetre of their course, only to break up into a tangle of fine beaded axons ending in poorly formed end-plates.

Another condition in which the terminal intramuscular innervation shows characteristic changes is the neuropathy seen in adult coeliac disease (Cooke, Johnson and Woolf, 1966). The terminal axonic expansions of the end-plates can be demonstrated in vitally-stained preparations to show marked swelling and fusion, a change rarely seen in any other condition. Conventional microscopy of muscle in this disease may show no abnormalities.

Myasthenia Gravis

Myasthenia gravis is a distinctive muscle disease, the main clinical feature of which is the development of muscle weakness following activity. Recovery occurs after a period of inactivity. The condition has attracted much attention and a voluminous literature, beginning with a description of a case by Thomas Willis (1672). There is an excellent review of the early literature by Campbell and Bramwell (1900). A recent account of the disease is that by Simpson (1969). The condition is

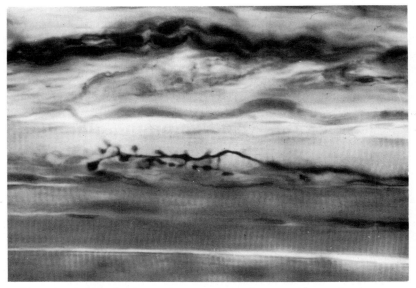

Figure 3–11 Myasthenia gravis. Posterior cricoarytenoid muscle (laryngectomy specimen) showing enlargement of the motor-end plate. (Schofield, ×520.)

considered here because it is thought that the neuromuscular apparatus is the anatomical region principally involved.

The pathology of the muscle in myasthenia gravis was described by Weigert (1901) and Buzzard (1905), but a more recent account is that of Russell (1953). Russell, in a series of eight cases of myasthenia gravis, described three types of histological change. Type I was an acute change in which the muscle fibres underwent necrosis, with resulting inflammatory reaction and finally disappearance of the necrotic fibres. Type II was a progressive atrophy of individual fibres; this change, when extensive, was associated with the formation of lymphorrhages. Type III was atrophy of single fibres or groups of fibres.

The development of techniques of staining the motor nerve endings led to the discovery that the neuromuscular apparatus is abnormal in myasthenia gravis (Coërs and Desmedt, 1959). The synaptic plate is enlarged, with terminal knobs forming a very elongated end-plate region (Fig. 3–11). These changes are reviewed by Woolf (1969).

PATHOLOGY OF DENERVATION AS SEEN IN DISEASE

The reaction of the whole muscle and of the individual muscle fibres to denervation has been dealt with in detail in Chapter 2. What will be discussed here is the diagnostic value of the morphological changes of denervation that can be observed in the skeletal muscle. Emphasis will be placed on certain features of diagnostic assistance and factors which are important in interpretation of a muscle biopsy.

Motor Unit Atrophy

This name is given to a pattern of muscle fibre atrophy that is characteristic of denervation. In this pattern one sees groups of similarly atrophied muscle fibres among muscle fibres of normal sizes. These groups may consist of small or large numbers of muscle fibres; other areas may show scattered single atrophied muscle fibres. Although this histological feature seen in denervated muscle in biopsies and necropsies is constantly used in the recognition of denervating muscle diseases, the term motor unit atrophy requires some comment.

Our knowledge of the group of muscle fibres (up to 40) supplied by one neurone (the motor unit) allows us to visualise the result of the destruction of one neurone cell body and of the nerve fibres arising from this cell body. We know that the muscle fibres in the motor unit are grouped together but are not adjacent, because other fibres of nearby motor units are interspersed. This means that when one neurone degenerates, the group of muscle fibres picked out by the neurogenic atrophy are close together but not adjacent as a circumscribed group of muscle fibres. This normal arrangement is complicated by the regeneration of nerve fibres and the reinnervation of the denervated muscle fibres. A muscle fibre deprived of its innervation will, if possible, gain innervation from new sprouting branches of a neighbouring nerve fibre. This reinnervation happens on a large scale in a slowly progressive neuronal degeneration because in this type of disease there is time for the muscle fibres to regain a nerve supply before they degenerate. The reinnervation causes a change in the grouping of muscle fibres in the motor unit, which may enlarge and be made up of muscle fibres which are now closer together. Finally, if the motor neurone supplying this larger re-formed unit degenerates, there is atrophy of many muscle fibres arranged close together. This atrophy of closely packed muscle fibres is often called *motor unit atrophy* but would be more correctly termed *group fibre atrophy*.

Progressive Denervation Changes

It is usually possible to detect the changes of progressive denervation when these are present in a muscle biopsy, and the feature to look for is the varying size of the atrophying muscle fibres, which indicates varying stages of denervation. The most common condition causing this progressive denervation is motor neurone disease, and the detection of this change is an important aid to diagnosis. The converse of this useful marker is that an old region of denervated muscle fibres caused, for example, by acute poliomyelitis or by peripheral nerve trauma can be identified by the similarity in the stage of atrophy of all of the denervated muscle fibres.

Site of the Lower Motor Neurone Denervation

It is doubtful that we can distinguish from the morphological changes in the muscle whether the denervation is caused by a lesion of the spinal cord, or whether the primary location of the disease process is in the spinal nerve roots or in the peripheral nerve trunks. Denervation atrophy of the muscles concerned is common to all these disease patterns, and may also be seen in degeneration of intramuscular nerves and even in myasthenia gravis, where there is a physiological block at the motor end-plate. Other associated features are, however, often of help in distinguishing the location of denervation. Spinal cord disease may cause long tract degeneration of motor and sensory functions. Spinal nerve root disorders are characterised by pain as a symptom, while C.S.F. protein levels may be high. In peripheral nerve trunk disorders there is usually a combined motor and sensory neuropathy; in these cases a nerve biopsy (e.g., of the sural nerve) may give valuable additional information. In all cases the detailed anatomy of the denervation will point to the anatomical location of the denervating process.

Chronicity of Denervating Changes

The degree of the muscle fibre atrophy induced by denervation is a good index of the duration of the disease or process causing the denervation. In this way we can distinguish a very chronic denervating disease, such as peroneal muscle atrophy, from diseases causing subacute denervation. This distinction is often important in diagnosis, although the changes looked for are non-specific and are dependent on the time scale of the disease rather than on any inherent differences in the pathology.

Normal Appearance of Muscle in Denervation

An occasional finding is an apparently normal muscle biopsy obtained from a patient with a profound lower motor neurone weakness. There are three possible explanations for this paradox.

Firstly, the nerve lesion may be predominately one in which there is demyelination of the peripheral nerves, an example being Guillain-

Barré disease. In cases of this disease, profound flaccid paralysis may be present and yet the muscle shows apparently normal muscle fibres. Sometimes examination of the fine motor nerve endings will show degeneration, but even this may not be conspicuous.

Secondly, there may be a massive, near-complete destruction of motor neurones, as seen in anterior poliomyelitis in its acute stage and in the rapidly progressive forms of Werdnig-Hoffmann disease. The muscle biopsy in these cases shows no obvious disparity of muscle fibre size, because *all* of the muscle fibres are undergoing atrophy. Measurement of many muscle fibres and comparison of the figures with measurements made on control muscles (often difficult in a child) will confirm the widespread slight atrophy. Electron microscopy can also be used to demonstrate that the apparently normal muscle fibres are undergoing changes of denervation. Examination of the intramuscular nerve endings by silver or methylene blue techniques will show nerve degeneration.

Thirdly, the denervation may be too recent for the changes of denervation to be apparent as atrophy of muscle fibres. Examination of the small intramuscular nerve fibres may then show degeneration, as this change precedes the atrophic changes in the muscle fibre.

Upper Motor Neurone Lesions

It might be thought that there are no morphological changes to be seen in muscles made weak by an upper motor neurone lesion. However, study of such muscles has revealed minor but important changes. Human muscle contains approximately equal numbers of type I and type II muscle fibres, each being distinguished by a difference in biochemical enzymes corresponding to differences in action. Generally speaking, the type I fibres are concerned with the muscle tone used in the maintenance of posture, whereas type II fibres are used for sudden purposive movements. In upper motor neurone paralysis, purposive movements are abolished by the paralysis but postural tone is increased. Consequently, type II fibres atrophy while type I fibres show slight hypertrophy, and this causes a reversal in the size distinction. Type I fibres are normally smaller than type II fibres, but in muscles subjected to upper motor neurone paresis the reverse is the case.

References

Bowden, R. E. M. (1952). Some recent studies of skeletal muscle in anterior poliomyelitis and other neuromuscular disorders in man and the experimental animal. Poliomyelitis: papers and discussion presented at the 2nd International Conference, pp. 95–99. Lippincott, Philadelphia.

Buzzard, E. F. (1905). The clinical history and postmortem examination of five cases of myasthenia gravis. Brain *28*, 438–483.

Campbell, H., and Bramwell, E. (1900). Myasthenia gravis. Brain *23*, 277–336.

Coërs, C., and Desmedt, J. E. (1959). Mise en évidence d'une malformation caractéristique de la jonction neuromusculaire dans la myasthénie. Acta neurol. psychiat. belg. 59, 539–561.

Cooke, W. T., Johnson, A. G., and Woolf, A. L. (1966). Vital staining and electron microscopy of the intramuscular nerve endings in the neuropathy of adult coeliac disease. Brain 89, 663–682.

Drachman, D. B., Murphy, S. R., Nigam, M. P., and Hills, J. R. (1967). "Myopathic" changes in chronically denervated muscle. Arch. Neurol. 16, 14–24.

Gardner-Medwin, D., and Walton, J. N. (1969). A classification of the neuromuscular disorders and a note on the clinical examination of the voluntary muscles. In Disorders of Voluntary Muscle. 2nd ed. J. N. Walton, (ed.). Churchill, London.

Hughes, J.T. (1966). Pathology of the Spinal Cord. Lloyd-Luke, London.

Hughes, J. T., and Brownell, B. (1964). Cervical spondylosis complicated by anterior spinal artery thrombosis. Neurology (Minneap.) 14,1073–1077.

Hughes, J. T., and Brownell, B. (1969). Ultrastructure of muscle in Werdnig-Hoffmann disease. J. neurol. Sci. 8, 363–379.

Russell, D. S. (1953). Histological changes in the striped muscles in myasthenia gravis. J. Path. Bact. 65, 279–289.

Simpson, J. A. (1969). Myasthenia gravis and myasthenic syndromes. In Disorders of Voluntary Muscle. 2nd ed. J. N. Walton, (Ed.). Churchill, London.

Weigert, C. (1901). Pathologisch-anatomischer Beitrag zur Erb'schen Krankheit (Myasthenia Gravis). Neurol. Zbl. (Leipzig) 20, 597–601.

Woolf, A. L. (1969). Pathological anatomy of the intramuscular nerve endings. In Disorders of Voluntary Muscle. 2nd ed. J. N. Walton. (Ed.). Churchill, London.

Chapter Four

Muscle Dystrophies

Although the muscular dystrophies form a well-recognised group of diseases, there is difficulty in their exact definition. Walton (Walton and Gardner-Medwin, 1969) has defined a muscular dystrophy as a *progressive, genetically determined, primary, degenerative myopathy,* and it is helpful to examine the components of this definition.

Myopathy, as used in this textbook, means only a disorder of muscle, and essentially a muscle dystrophy is a *degenerative* myopathy caused by some defect located, as far as we know, within the muscle fibre *(primary).* This elaboration of our definition avoids including periodic paralysis and McArdle's syndrome among the dystrophies. Probably all muscular dystrophies are *genetically determined,* and the exceptions seen as sporadic cases can be explained by our knowledge of the expression of genetic characteristics. *Progressive* degeneration of the muscle fibre is always present in muscle dystrophy, and is not seen in some benign myopathies that otherwise might be regarded as dystrophies.

The various classifications of muscular dystrophies are based on clinical and genetic differences, and either of these features may be emphasised. The accounts of Levison (1951), Stevenson (1953), Becker (1953), Walton and Nattrass (1954), Walton (1955) and Dubowitz (1965) show the development of our modern classification. For our purpose here, the dystrophies will be classified on clinical and genetic grounds into four groups: (1) *Duchenne dystrophy* (sex-linked recessive); (2) *limb-girdle dystrophy* (autosomal recessive); (3) *facioscapulohumeral dystrophy* (autosomal dominant); and (4) *dystrophia myotonica* (autosomal dominant). For an account of the many other rarer forms of dystrophy the reader is referred to Bourne and Golarz (1962), and Walton and Gardner-Medwin (1969).

DUCHENNE DYSTROPHY

Duchenne dystrophy, also called pseudohypertrophic dystrophy, is the commonest severe dystrophy and was the earliest described (Duchenne, 1868; Gowers, 1879).

This condition is inherited as a sex-linked recessive condition and appears almost invariably in males, who usually manifest the disease before the fifth year. Sporadic cases in young males presumed due to mutations are common. Two case reports of the disease in girls, who also suffered from Turner's syndrome, have been described (Walton, 1956; Ferrier, Bamatter and Klein, 1965). Instances of the disease in females (Dubowitz, 1960) are probably manifestations of the expression of the recessive gene in the carrier state.

The invariable course of the disease is the gradual development of weakness seen in the clinical setting of the developing child. Usually there is delay in standing and walking, but sometimes these milestones are achieved normally but followed by regression. The weakness begins in the large muscles of the pelvic and shoulder girdles. Inability to climb stairs and to rise from the floor is characteristic: Gowers (1879) first described the method often adopted of rising from the ground by using the arm muscles to raise the trunk above the legs. The weakness of the muscles is associated with hypotonia and hyporeflexia. The affected muscles are sometimes enlarged (pseudohypertrophy), and this frequently affects the calf muscles and sometimes the quadriceps or deltoid muscles. The weakness of muscle groups leads to contractures, skeletal wasting and deformity (Walton and Warrick, 1954). The weakness is steadily progressive, leading to inability to walk and finally death, which occurs in the second or third decade. Cardiac involvement is always present (Berenbaum and Horowitz, 1956) and is the usual cause of death, which otherwise is caused by respiratory infection. Moderate intellectual impairment occurs (Dubowitz, 1965; Rosman and Kakulas, 1966).

A benign form of sex-linked recessive muscular dystrophy, arising in adolescence and with a much slower progression, has been called the Becker type (Becker and Keiner, 1955; Becker, 1962). In this form cardiac involvement is rare; many of the late features of dystrophy may not develop, and a normal life span is possible. The only difference of this Becker subgroup is the mildness of the disease, and it has been suggested that the same gene may be responsible but with a difference in penetration. The mildness of the disease permits the affected males to reproduce and transmit the disease through their unaffected daughters to male grandchildren.

LIMB-GIRDLE DYSTROPHY

Walton (1962) has emphasised the distinctive features of limb-girdle dystrophy. The condition is usually transmitted by an autosomal recessive gene, but some examples of dominant inheritance are known. Sporadic examples are common and cause diagnostic difficulty. The development of the disease is very variable, but the commonest time of onset is after the second decade, with a relatively benign course but causing serious debility after about 20 years. Some cases are very mild in character and in others the progress of the disease seems to be arrested with little further deterioration.

The distribution of the muscle weakness characteristically affects the large muscles of the shoulder and pelvic girdles, but even this feature is variable. In some cases only one or two muscles (e.g., the quadriceps or vastus medialis) are affected at first, and only after many years are the limb-girdle muscles involved. Pseudohypertrophy of the affected muscles is seen in some but not all cases. There are usually no bony deformities or joint contractures until the patient is confined to bed. The heart is usually not involved and there is no mental deterioration.

FACIOSCAPULOHUMERAL MUSCULAR DYSTROPHY

This condition is also called after Landouzy and Déjèrine (1884), who gave a good description of the disease. The inheritance is predominately by an autosomal dominant gene and consequently the disease occurs in either sex, the age of onset varying from late childhood to adult life. The severity of the illness is very variable, but most cases are benign. Subclinical cases are common in an affected family and will only be found by a survey of relatives of a definite case. The course of the disease is that of the slow development of weakness, sometimes with arrest of the progression of the disease. There is a sequential involvement of the muscles of the face, shoulder girdle and pelvic girdle. Sometimes the facial involvement is slight, and these cases can be confused with cases of limb-girdle dystrophy. The life expectancy of patients with this disease is not necessarily shortened. There is rarely any pseudohypertrophy, and bony changes and joint contractures do not occur. There is no cardiac involvement or cerebral degeneration.

DYSTROPHIA MYOTONICA

Dystrophia myotonica is the best known of the myotonic disorders, in which group are included Thomsen's disease or myotonia congenita (Thomsen, 1876) and paramyotonia congenita (Eulenberg, 1886). It is not yet clear whether these three conditions are separate diseases or different clinical manifestations of the same disease. There have been very few reports of the pathological changes in Thomsen's disease or in paramyotonia congenita, and further study of the pathological changes in all cases with increased muscular tone is required. A good review is the account of Thomasen (1948).

In contrast to myotonia congenita and paramyotonia congenita, dystrophia myotonica is frequently diagnosed, and the pathology of the changes in the muscle has been extensively studied (Thomasen, 1948; Caughey and Myrianthopoulos, 1963). The first descriptions of the disease were by Steinert (1909) and Batten and Gibb (1909).

The disease is a constellation of congenital abnormalities, of which the muscle weakness with myotonia concerns us here. The associated abnormalities are cataracts, baldness, gonadal atrophy, heart disease and dementia. The condition is inherited by an autosomal dominant gene and affected families are stricken with a profound disability.

The muscle weakness usually manifests itself in the limbs, with difficulty in walking and in using the hands. The myotonia is seen usually in the hands, and the grip cannot be easily relaxed. The muscles of the face and neck are affected by the weakness, causing an alteration in the facial expression. The disease is usually steadily progressive, with death occurring after about 20 years of the illness. The heart is usually involved and death by cardiac failure is common; otherwise the end is by a terminal bronchopneumonia. Dystrophia myotonica not only is distinguishable from other dystrophies clinically but has specific pathological changes in the muscles which will be described later.

Dystrophia myotonica in the first 5 years of life is a rare but important clinical variant of the disease. The affected child may have only facial weakness and dysphagia, and because the myotonia is difficult to detect the diagnosis is often difficult (Vanier, 1960; Pruzanski, 1966).

BIOCHEMICAL CHANGES IN MUSCLE DYSTROPHIES

The widespread metabolic disturbance caused by the extensive muscle necrosis in muscle dystrophy results in a large variety of biochemical changes. The most important and useful change is the elevation of certain enzymes in the blood, and this change will be described in some detail. Other biochemical changes will be more briefly mentioned. For a more detailed account the reader is referred to Pennington (1969).

Serum Enzymes

The levels of certain enzymes in the blood are markedly raised in muscle dystrophies. This finding is not specific, but appears to be due to leakage of the enzymes from the damaged muscle fibres. Despite the lack of specificity, these tests are of the greatest value, both in diagnosis and prognosis. With the exception of occasional cases of polymyositis, only in cases of the muscle dystrophies are very high values of serum enzyme levels obtained, and thus these very high values can be taken as strong evidence for the existence of a muscle dystrophy. The height of the serum enzyme levels also indicates the activity of the disease in a known case of dystrophy. In the early stages of Duchenne dystrophy the values are high, but later, as the amount of muscle still capable of degeneration dwindles, the levels are lower. In the last stages of the disease, when most of the muscle has been replaced by fibrous tissue and fat, the levels may be barely above normal. Elevation of serum enzymes occurs before any clinical manifestations of the disease (Pearson, 1957), and this phenomenon allows the diagnosis to be made soon after birth in a child who may not be demonstrably weak for some months or even years. The subclinical carrier state may also be diagnosed by the moderate elevation of serum enzyme levels in conjunction with other electrophysiological and pathological evidence. The two enzymes which currently are most frequently used in the diagnosis of muscle diseases are creatine-kinase and aldolase.

SERUM CREATINE-KINASE

The levels of serum creatine-kinase are of the most value in the diagnosis of dystrophy. Since the work of Ebashi, Toyokura, Momoi and Sugita (1959), it has been known that in muscle dystrophy there is a spectacular elevation of the serum levels of this enzyme. Pearce, Pennington and Walton (1964a, 1964b, 1964c) have made an exhaustive study of the levels of this enzyme in normal individuals and in many muscle and neuromuscular diseases. These authors have established normal values of up to 3.5 μ moles of creatine per hour per ml of serum, which figure is equivalent to 60 international units per litre. In the early stages of Duchenne dystrophy the values may be 500 times the normal value of 60 international units/litre. In the later stages of the disease the levels, although usually still high, diminish. In dystrophia myotonica and in the adult dystrophies, moderate increases are obtained. About two thirds of female carriers of Duchenne dystrophy show slight elevation of this serum enzyme.

SERUM ALDOLASE

The rise of this enzyme in the serum of cases of muscular dystrophy was discovered by Sibley and Lehninger (1949), and subsequently this finding has been confirmed by many workers (Dreyfus, Schapira and Schapira, 1958; Chung, Morton and Peters, 1960; Thomson, Leyburn and Walton, 1960). Normal values, expressed as Bruns units, are less than ten (Pennington, 1969). In Duchenne dystrophy there is a rise which may reach 100 units and the level indicates the activity of the disease. In the less active adult forms of dystrophy and in the late stages of Duchenne dystrophy the rise in serum aldolase is less. Normal levels are usually obtained in cases of neurogenic atrophy and myasthenia gravis. Occasionally in cases of rapidly progressive polymyositis high levels may be obtained, but apart from this disease a high level of serum aldolase indicates an active form of muscle dystrophy.

Other Biochemical Changes in Muscle Dystrophy

In muscle dystrophies and in other muscle diseases with rapid degeneration of the muscle fibre, there is an increase in the blood creatine and in the urinary creatine excretion. The excretion of some of the amino acids in the urine is also increased. Blood electrolytes appear to be normal in dystrophies. Of the serum proteins the α 2 globulin fraction is raised; this may be because of an increase in sialic acid which is present in this fraction and which has been shown to be elevated in dystrophy. Urinary excretion of myoglobin occurs in certain diseases in which there is destruction of the muscle fibres.

HISTOPATHOLOGY OF MUSCLE IN DYSTROPHIES

Except for dystrophia myotonica, the histopathological features of the muscle dystrophies will be described together. As far as we know, there are no specific histological changes that would allow us to distinguish the various clinical and genetic types of dystrophy. A wide range of pathological alterations may be found in different cases of dystrophy, in muscle from the same case at different stages of the disease, and even from different muscles from the same case examined at the same time. The range of changes is attributable to the rapidity of the disease process and the stage of the disease attained in the tissue examined. The following account of histopathological change is mainly from the author's personal experience, but has been amplified by the accounts of Erb (1884, 1891), Pick (1900), Wohlfahrt and Wohlfahrt (1935), Hassin (1943), Adams, Denny-Brown and Pearson (1962) and Adams (1969).

Macroscopical Appearance of the Muscles

At a surgical excision of muscle for biopsy the muscle usually looks abnormal, and the necropsy of a patient dying in the advanced stages of dystrophy shows striking changes in the muscles. The abnormalities consist of a change in colour to a greyish translucent appearance and in consistency to one which resembles fat rather than normal muscle. These changes in macroscopical appearance are due to the replacement of the muscles by fatty and fibrous tissue which, however, retains the form of the muscle and of its individual fascicles. The normal sub-units of the muscle are preserved, but fat has largely replaced the muscle fibres. Usually the muscles appear atrophied, but pseudohypertrophy is often seen in some muscles at some stages of the disease. The pseudohypertrophy consists of excess fatty and fibrous tissue which, for reasons which are not clear, occupies more bulk than the muscle it replaces.

Microscopical Appearance of the Muscles

The various histological changes seen in the muscle in dystrophy will be considered under the following headings: *loss of muscle fibres, fatty and fibrous tissue replacement, degeneration of muscle fibres, cytoplasmic changes in fibres* and *nuclear changes.*

LOSS OF MUSCLE FIBRES

The most striking feature in muscle dystrophy (except in the early stages, in mild cases, or in muscle groups less affected) is a profound loss of muscle fibres (Fig. 4–1). In advanced cases there may be only oc-

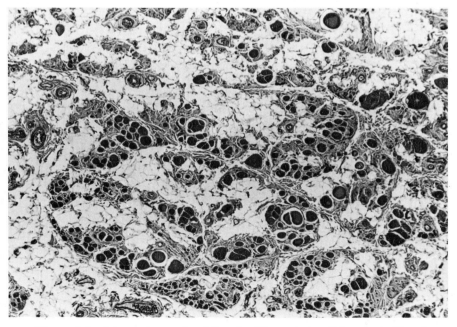

Figure 4–1 Advanced muscular dystrophy. The majority of the muscle fibres have degenerated and have been replaced by fat. (Haematoxylin and eosin, × 50.)

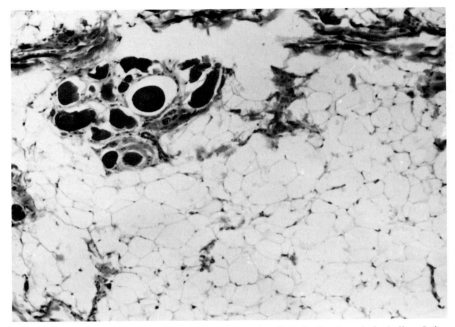

Figure 4-2   End stage of muscular dystrophy. Practically the whole belly of the muscle has been converted into fat. A search found only the small bundle of abnormal muscle fibres seen top left. (Haematoxylin and eosin, × 100).

casional muscle fibres present in a microscope field. This extensive loss of muscle fibres is most notable in the late stages of Duchenne dystrophy; in these cases fat and fibrous tissue form the bulk of the muscle belly, which now contains few muscle fibres. Pseudohypertrophic areas of muscle in the early stages probably consist of many large muscle fibres, but later the muscle becomes converted to connective tissue and fat (Fig. 4-2).

FAT AND FIBROUS TISSUE REPLACEMENT

Muscle fibres lost as the result of any muscle or neuromuscular disease are replaced by fatty and fibrous tissue. This happens not only in muscle dystrophies but also in cases of polymyositis and following acute denervation. It is common as a sequel of the denervation of poliomyelitis but is not seen in motor neurone disease, in which the time course is shorter. Fat and fibrous tissue replacement is marked in the late stages of Duchenne dystrophy, when all the muscle bellies become converted to fatty tissue. This fatty change is present in all dystrophies, but the degree varies from case to case.

DEGENERATION OF MUSCLE FIBRES

In all skeletal muscle examined from cases of severe muscular dys-trophy, a proportion of muscle fibres are undergoing degeneration, and this universal involvement of skeletal muscles is very helpful in making the diagnosis. The cytoplasm of the affected muscle fibres becomes granular and may be vacuolated (Fig. 4–3). The normal striations are lost and the myofibrils become disorganised. The sarcoplasm of the muscle fibre is gathered into homogenous masses, causing distention of the muscle fibre (Figs. 4–4 and 4–5). The cell fills with phagocytes, which ultimately absorb the breakdown products of the disintegrating cell (Fig. 4–6). The process of degeneration is relatively slow, which may explain why there is little inflammatory reaction. Exceptionally, when rapid degeneration of many adjacent muscle fibres occurs, an inflammatory reaction can be seen, and in these areas the appearance may lead to diag-nostic confusion with polymyositis. Except for the occasional occurrence of this minor degree of inflammation, the absence of acute inflammation is an important diagnostic observation, distinguishing the degeneration of dystrophy from that of polymyositis.

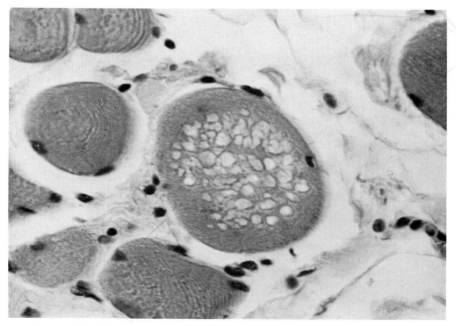

Figure 4–3 Muscular dystrophy. Vacuolar degeneration in a muscle fibre seen in transverse section. (Haematoxylin and eosin, × 300).

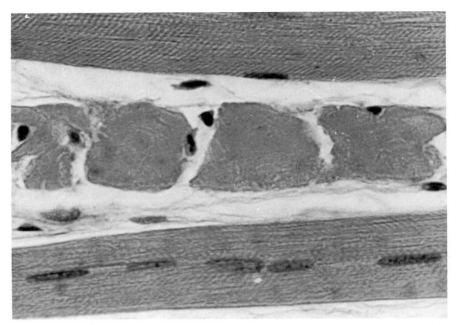

Figure 4–4   Same case as in Figure 4–3. The picture shows a degenerating muscle fibre seen in longitudinal section. (Haematoxylin and eosin, × 300).

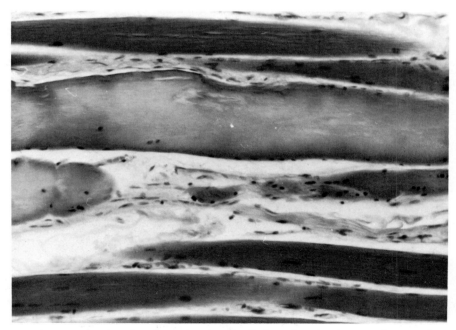

Figure 4–5   Muscular dystrophy. Longitudinal section showing two degenerating muscle fibres. (Haematoxylin and eosin, × 250).

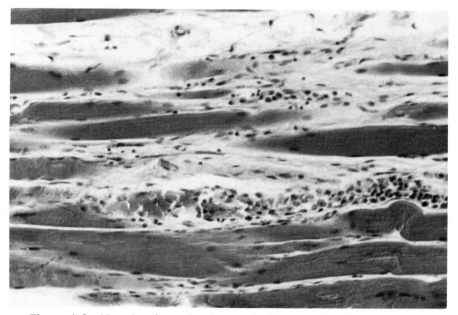

Figure 4-6 Muscular dystrophy. Longitudinal section showing a degenerating muscle fibre filled with phagocytes. (Haematoxylin and eosin, × 200).

CYTOPLASMIC CHANGES IN MUSCLE FIBRES

In the majority of muscle fibres changes of degeneration are not seen, and yet there are important abnormalities of size and shape (Figs. 4–7 and 4–8). The other feature that is usually present is the presence of "daughter" muscle fibres (Fig. 4–9); the absence of features of regeneration is another important observation.

Variation in size of muscle fibres is an important finding in muscle dystrophy and a helpful point when one is confronted with an otherwise doubtful muscle biposy. Size variation is not only present in muscles that are affected clinically; it may also be apparent in muscles that are clinically normal. It can sometimes be seen in the muscle of close relatives who have a subclinical carrier state. The usual finding is a random distribution of abnormally small or abnormally large muscle fibres. The small fibres are more numerous but it is the large ones that are striking, since they may be up to 250 μ in diameter; the small fibres may be as small as 10 μ in diameter (Figs. 4–7 and 4–8).

The abnormally sized fibres are usually much rounder than normal or denervated muscle fibres, and this is an important distinctive feature separating dystrophy from denervation. In denervating diseases, abnormally small muscle fibres are a constant finding, but these are usually *more, not less,* angular.

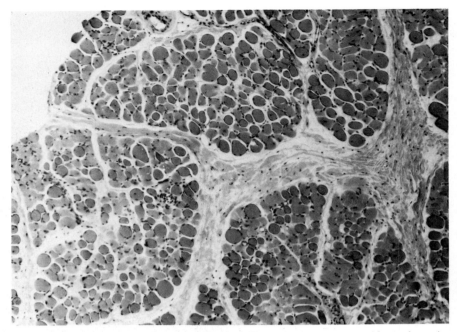

Figure 4–7 Muscular dystrophy. Early changes seen in sternomastoid muscle cut in transverse section. The muscle fibres are not seriously depleted but many are abnormal. The muscle fibres are rounded and their size is variable. The sarcolemmal nuclei are increased and often centrally placed. (Haematoxylin and eosin, ×50).

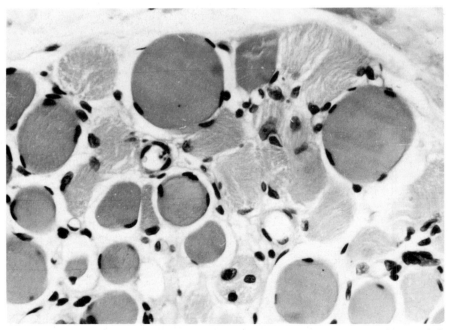

Figure 4–8 High power view of part of picture seen in Figure 4–1. Note the rounded muscle fibres of uneven size. There are degenerating fibres with centrally placed nuclei. (Haematoxylin and eosin, ×250).

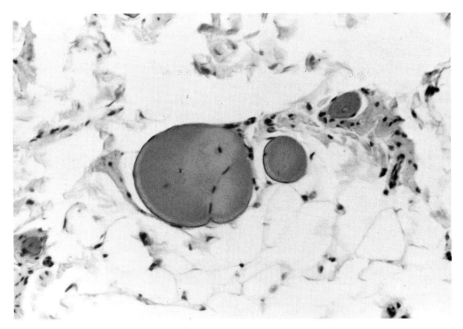

Figure 4–9   Muscular dystrophy. Transverse section of muscle fibre which is splitting into two "daughter" muscle fibres. (Haematoxylin and eosin, × 250).

Finally, the abnormally large muscle fibres are frequently observed dividing into two, three or four daughter fibres (Fig. 4–9). This feature is not usually seen in any condition except dystrophy.

NUCLEAR CHANGES IN THE MUSCLE FIBRES

In normal muscle, sarcolemmal nuclei are present in moderate numbers and are peripherally situated, but in muscle dystrophy there is an increase in the number of nuclei, which are often centrally placed. This finding is frequently seen in severe childhood dystrophies but is also prominent in dystrophia myotonica. However, these nuclear changes are not specific to dystrophy. They occur in polymyositis and in regenerating muscle due to other causes.

Dystrophia Myotonica

There are distinctive histological features in the muscle of cases of dystrophia myotonica that must be added to those already described in the other dystrophies. These features are muscle fibre hypertrophy, nuclear abnormalities, sarcoplasmic masses, ringbinden, and distortion of fibre structures. Muscle fibre hypertrophy is common, but measurement of fibres may be required for its demonstration. Large numbers of small, centrally placed sarcolemmal nuclei are another feature of dystrophia myotonica. Long chains of central nuclei, if trauma to the muscle can be excluded, are also very suggestive of the condition. Sarcoplasmic masses are large, longitudinally oriented, elongated masses of densely staining sarcoplasm without myofibrils. They may occupy up to two thirds of the cross sectional area of fibres. Central nuclei are particularly prominent in muscle dystrophies and are most numerous in dystrophia myotonica.

ULTRASTRUCTURAL STUDIES

Despite a great deal of study, the ultrastructure of the degenerating muscle fibre in dystrophy has not yet revealed differences peculiar to dystrophy and absent from other degenerative muscle conditions. It has also been found that the disorganisation of the muscle fibre following denervation has many features in common with the degeneration of the muscle fibre in muscle dystrophy.

Ultrastructure of Muscle in Cases of Dystrophy

The following papers contain accounts of the ultrastructural changes in muscle dystrophies: Mölbert (1960), Van Breemen (1960), Lapresle, Fardeau and Milhaud (1966), Fisher, Cohn and Danowski (1966), Hudgson, Pearce and Walton (1967), Santa (1969), Mastaglia, Papadimitriou and Kakulas (1970) and Mair and Tomé (1972).

The ultrastructural changes found differ markedly according to the stage of the disease (Figs. 4–10 to 4–12). In the early stages and in biopsies from patients at a preclinical stage there is a moderate loss of myofilaments from the periphery of the sarcomeres; this change results in a widening of the intermyofibrillar spaces (Fig. 4–11). A later change is disarray of the band structure, which affects the I bands more than the Z lines (Fig. 4–12). The sarcoplasm appears to be increased, and mitochondria are often numerous. Glycogen may be abundant. The tubular system is often prominent and is probably greatly enlarged, although of irregular form. The changes just described refer to the abnormally large muscle fibres, but many muscle fibres are smaller than normal. These atrophied fibres have lost most of their sarcomeres but often retain their sarcolemmal nuclei, which appear increased and may be centrally placed. The basement membrane of the muscle cell does not atrophy, and appears as redundant folds. Part of the abnormal histological picture in dystrophy is the appearance of adventitial cells, many of which are phagocytes within the degenerating muscle fibres. Fibroblasts are

(Text continued on page 90.)

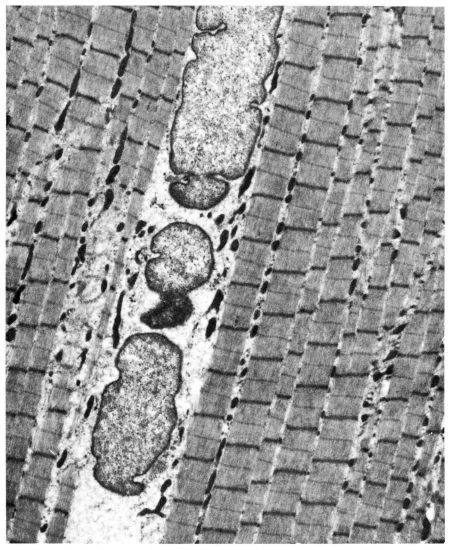

Figure 4–10 Muscular dystrophy. Electron micrograph of a longitudinal section of a muscle fibre showing early changes. Many central nuclei are present. (Phosphotungstic acid, × 8000).

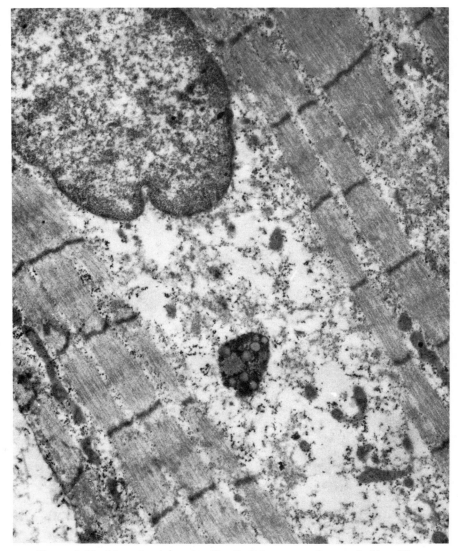

Figure 4–11 Muscular dystrophy. Detail of the centre of a muscle fibre. The myofibrils have lost myofilaments with widening of the intermyofibrillar space which contains a lysosome. (Phosphotungstic acid, × 14,000.)

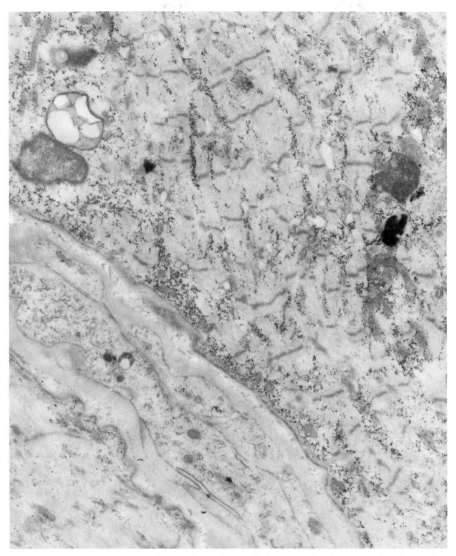

Figure 4–12   Muscular dystrophy. Advanced degeneration in a muscle fibre. The photomicrograph shows disorganisation of the band structure with lysosomes and lipid droplets. (2% uranyl acetate and lead citrate, × 7000.)

increased in number, and in the advanced stages of the disease there are many collagen fibres. Inflammatory cells are uncommon, except when the disease is at its most active stage. Satellite cells may be found either in relation to degenerating muscle fibres or related to normal muscle fibres.

Ultrastructural Changes in the Carrier State

Electron microscopy has been used in the examination of the muscle of possible carriers of dystrophy to search for changes which might indicate the carrier state. Relevant observations have been made by Milhorat, Shafiq and Goldstone (1966), Roy and Dubowitz (1970) and Beckmann, Kloke and Freund-Mölbert (1970). Ultrastructural changes have been found and considered to be abnormal in many persons proved to be carriers. However, at the present time the changes that have been found are thought to be non-specific. Evidence of the carrier state from ultrastructural changes should be considered in conjunction with light microscopical findings and with the changes in the serum enzyme levels.

Ultrastructural Changes in Dystrophia Myotonica

There have been several reports of the ultrastructural changes of the muscle in dystrophia myotonica, and the following is a selection of the accounts available: Wechsler and Hager (1961), Aleu and Afifi (1964), Klinkerfuss (1967), Schroeder and Adams (1968), and Schotland (1970).

Changes similar to those in other dystrophies have been found, but in addition, the "ringbinden" and sarcoplasmic masses familiar in light microscopy have been further studied.

References

Adams, R. D. (1969). *In* Disorders of Voluntary Muscle. J. N. Walton (Ed.). Churchill, London.

Adams, R. D., Denny-Brown, D., and Pearson, C. M. (1962). Diseases of Muscle: A Study in Pathology. 2nd ed. Hoeber, New York.

Adie, W. J., and Greenfield, J. G. (1923). Dystrophia myotonica (myotonia atrophica). Brain *46*, 73–127.

Aleu, F. P., and Afifi, A. K. (1964). Ultrastructure of muscles in myotonic dystrophy. Preliminary observations. Amer. J. Path. *45*, 221–231.

Allen, J. E., and Rodgin, D. W. (1960). Mental retardation in association with progressive muscular dystrophy. A.M.A. J. Dis. Child. *100*, 208–211.

Aran, F. A. (1850). Recherches sur une maladie non encore décrite du système musculaire (atrophie musculaire progressive). Arch. gén. Méd. *24*, 5.

Banker, B. Q., Victor, M., and Adams, R. D. (1957). Arthrogryposis multiplex due to congenital muscular dystrophy. Brain *80*, 319–334.

Batten, F. E. (1903). Three cases of myopathy, infantile type. Brain *26*, 147–148.

Batten, F. E., and Gibb, H. P. (1909). Myotonia atrophica. Brain *32*, 187–205.

Becker, P. E. (1953). Dystrophia Musculorum Progressiva. Thieme, Stuttgart.

Becker, P. E. (1962). Two new families of benign sex-linked recessive muscular dystrophy. Rev. Canad. Biol. *21*, 551–566.

Becker, P. E., and Keiner, F. (1955). Eine neue x-chromosomale Muskeldystrophie. Arch. Psychiat. (Berlin) *193*, 427–428.

Beckmann, R., Kloke, W. D., and Freund-Mölbert, E. R. G. (1970). Ultrastructural findings in "carriers" of Duchenne muscular dystrophy. *In* Proc. Int. Cong. Muscle Disease, Milan, 1969. Walton, J. N., Canal, N., and Scarlato, G. (Eds.). Int. Cong. Ser. No. 199, pp. 439–444. Excerpta Medica, Amsterdam.

Berenbaum, A. A., and Horowitz, W. (1956). Heart involvement in progressive muscular dystrophy, report of a case with sudden death. Amer. Heart J. *51*, 622–627.

Bourne, G. H., and Golarz, N. (1962). Muscular Dystrophy in Man and Animals. Karger, Basel & New York.

Caughey, J. E., and Myrianthopoulos, N. C. (1963). Dystrophia myotonica and related disorders. Charles C Thomas, Springfield, Illinois.

Chung, C. S., Morton, N. E., and Peters, H. A. (1960). Serum enzymes and genetic carriers in muscular dystrophy. Amer. J. Hum. Genet. *12*, 52–66.

Church, S. C. (1967). The heart in myotonia atrophica. Arch. Intern. Med. *119*, 176–181.

Dreyfus, J. C., Schapira, G., and Schapira, F. (1958). Serum enzymes in the physiopathology of muscle. Ann. N.Y. Acad. Sci. *75*, 235.

Dubowitz, V. (1960). Progressive muscular dystrophy of the Duchenne type in females and its mode of inheritance. Brain *83*, 432–439.

Dubowitz, V. (1965). Intellectual impairment in muscular dystrophy. Arch. Dis. Child. *40*, 296–301.

Duchenne, G. B. (1868). Recherches sur la paralysie musculaire pseudo-hypertrophique ou paralysie myosclerosique. Arch. gén. Méd. *11*, 5, 179, 305, 421, 552.

Ebashi, S., Toyokura, Y., Momoi, H., and Sugita, H. (1959). High creatine phosphokinase activity of sera of progressive muscular dystrophy patients. J. Biochem. (Tokyo) *46*, 103.

Emery, A. E. H., Clack, E. R., Simon, S., and Taylor, J. L. (1967). Detection of carriers of benign x-linked muscular dystrophy. Brit. Med. J. *4*, 522–523.

Erb, W. H. (1884). Ueber die "juvenile Form" der progressiven Muskelatrophie ihre Beziehungen zur sogennanten Pseudohypertrophie der Muskeln. Dtsch. Arch. klin. Med. *34*, 467–519.

Erb, W. H. (1891). Dystrophia muscularis progressiva. Klinische und pathologisch-anatomische Studien. Dtsch. Z. Nervenheilkd. *1*, 13–94, 173–261.

Eulenberg, A. (1886). Ueber eine familiäre, durch 6 generationen verfolgbare Form congenitaler Paramyotonie. Neurol. Zbl. (Leipzig) *5*, 265–272.

Ferrier, P., Bamatter, F., and Klein, D. (1965). Muscular dystrophy (Duchenne) in a girl with Turner's syndrome. J. Med. Genet. *2*, 38–46.

Fisch, C. (1951). The heart in dystrophia myotonica. Amer. Heart J. *41*, 525–538.

Fisher, E. R., Cohn, R. E., and Danowski, T. S. (1966). Ultrastructural observations of skeletal muscle in myopathy and neuropathy with special reference to muscular dystrophy. Lab. Invest. *15*, 778–793.

Gowers, W. R. (1879). Pseudohypertrophic Muscular Paralysis. Churchill, London.

Greenfield, J. G., Cornman, T., and Shy, G. M. (1958). The prognostic value of the muscle biopsy in the "floppy infant." Brain *81*, 461–484.

Hassin, G. B. (1943). The histopathology of progressive muscular dystrophy. J. Neuropath. Exp. Neurol. *2*, 315–325.

Hudgson, P., Pearce, G. W., and Walton, J. N. (1967). Preclinical muscular dystrophy: histopathological changes observed on muscle biopsy. Brain *90*, 565–576.

Jackson, C. E., and Carey, J. H. (1961). Progressive muscular dystrophy: autosomal recessive type. Paediatrics *28*, 77–84.

Jacobs, K. (1968). Carrier detection in the Duchenne type muscular dystrophy: preliminary observations on the place of electromyography. J. neurol. Sci. *6*, 347–356.

Klinkerfuss, G. H. (1967). An electron microscopic study of myotonic dystrophy. Arch. Neurol. *16*, 181–193.

Kugelberg, E., and Welander, L. (1956). Heredofamilial juvenile muscular atrophy simulating muscular dystrophy. Arch. Neurol. Psychiat. *75*, 500–509.

Landouzy, L., and Déjèrine, J. (1885). De la myopathie atrophique progressive; myopathie sans neuropathie, débutant d'ordinaire dans l'enfance, par la face. Rev. de Méd. *5*, 81–117; 253–366.

Lapresle, J., Fardeau, M., and Milhaud, M. (1966). Etude des ultrastructures dans les dystrophies musculaires progressives. Proc. 5th Int. Cong. Neuropath., pp. 602–603. Excerpta Medica, Amsterdam.

Levison, H. (1951). Dystrophia musculorum progressiva. Ejnor Munksgaards. Forlag., Copenhagen.

Mair, W. G. P., and Tomé, F. M. S. (1972). Atlas of the Ultrastructure of Diseased Human Muscle. Churchill Livingstone, Edinburgh & London.

Mastaglia, F. L., Papadimitriou, J. M., and Kakulas, B. A. (1970). Regeneration of muscle in Duchenne muscular dystrophy: an electron microscopy study. J. neurol. Sci. *11*, 425–444.

Milhorat, A. T., Shafiq, S. A., and Goldstone, L. (1966). Changes in muscle structure in dystrophic patients, carriers and normal siblings seen by electron microscopy: correlation with levels of serum creatinophosphokinase (CPK). Ann. N.Y. Acad. Sci. *138*, 246–292.

Mölbert, E. (1960). Das elecktronenmikroskopische Bild des Skeletmuskels bei Dystrophia musculorum progressiva Erb. Naturwissenschaften *47*, 186–187.

Nevin, S. (1936). Two cases of muscular degeneration occurring in late adult life, with a review of the recorded cases of late progressive muscular dystrophy (late progressive myopathy). Quart. J. Med. *5*, 51–68.

Pearce, G. W., Pearce, J. M. S., and Walton, J. N. (1966). The Duchenne type muscular dystrophy: histopathological studies of the carrier state. Brain *89*, 109–120.

Pearce, J. M. S., Pennington, R. J., and Walton, J. N. (1964a). Serum enzyme studies in muscle disease. I. Variations in serum creatine kinase activity in normal individuals. J. Neurol. Neurosurg. Psychiat. *27*, 1–4.

Pearce, J. M. S., Pennington, R. J., and Walton, J. N. (1964b). Serum enzyme studies in muscle disease. II. Serum creatine kinase activity in muscular dystrophy and in other myopathic and neuropathic disorders. J. Neurol. Neurosurg. Psychiat. *27*, 96–99.

Pearce, J. M. S., Pennington, R. J., and Walton, J. N. (1964c). Serum enzyme studies in muscle disease. III. Serum creatine kinase activity in relatives of patients with the Duchenne type of muscular dystrophy. J. Neurol. Neurosurg. Psychiat. *27*, 181–185.

Pearson, C. M. (1957). Serum enzymes in muscular dystrophy and certain other muscular and neuromuscular diseases. I. Serum glutamic oxalacetic transaminase. New Eng. J. Med. *256*, 1069–1075.

Pennington, R. J. (1969). Biochemical aspects of muscle disease. *In* Disorders of Voluntary Muscle. J. N. Walton (Ed.). Churchill, London.

Pick, F. (1900). Zur. Kenntnis der progressiven Muskelatrophie. Dtsch. Z. Nervenheilkd. *17*, 1–56.

Pruzanski, W. (1966). Variants of myotonic dystrophy in pre-adolescent life (the syndrome of myotonic dysembryoplasia). Brain *89*, 563–568.

Rosman, N. P., and Kakulas, B. A. (1966). Mental deficiency associated with muscular dystrophy. A neuropathological study. Brain *89*, 769–788.

Roy, S., and Dubowitz, V. (1970). Carrier detection in Duchenne muscular dystrophy. A comparative study of electron microscopy, light microscopy and serum enzymes. J. neurol. Sci. *11*, 65–79.

Santa, T. (1969). Fine structure of the human skeletal muscle in myopathy. Arch. Neurol. *20*, 479–489.

Schotland, D. L. (1970). An electron microscopic investigation of myotonic dystrophy: J. Neuropath. Exp. Neurol. *29*, 241–253.

Schroeder, J. M., and Adams, R. D. (1968). The ultrastructural morphology of the muscle fibres in myotonic dystrophy. Acta neuropath. *10*, 218–241.

Sibley, J. A., and Lehninger, A. L. (1949). Determination of aldolase in animal tissues. J. Biol. Chem. *177*, 859–872.

Smith, H. L., Amick, L. D., and Johnson, W. W. (1966). Detection of subclinical and carrier states in Duchenne muscular dystrophy. J. Pediat. *69*, 67–79.

Steinert, H. (1909). Ueber das klinische und anatomische Bild des muskelschwundes der Myotoniker. Dtsch. Z. Nervenheilkd. *37*, 38–104.

Stephens, J., and Lewin, E. (1965). Serum enzyme variations and histological abnormalities in the carrier state in Duchenne dystrophy. J. Neurol. Neurosurg. Psychiat. *28*, 104–108.

Stevenson, A. C. (1953). Muscular dystrophy in Northern Ireland. Ann. Eugen. (London) *18*, 50.

Thomasen, E. (1948). Thomsen's Disease, Paramyotonia, Dystrophia Myotonica. Universitets forlaget, Aarhus.

Thompson, M. W., Murphy, E. G., and McAlpine, P. J. (1967). An assessment of the creatine kinase test in the detection of carriers of Duchenne muscular dystrophy. J. Pediat. *71*, 82–93.

Thomsen, J. (1876). Tonische krämpfe in wilkürlich beweglichen muskeln in folge von ererbter psychischer disposition (ataxia muscularis?) Arch. Psychiat. Nervenkr. *6*, 706.

Thomson, W. H. S., Leyburn, P., and Walton, J. N. (1960). Serum enzyme activity in muscular dystrophy. Brit. Med. J. *2*, 1276–1281.

Turner, J. W. A., and Lees, F. (1962). Congenital myopathy—a fifty-year follow-up. Brain *85*, 733–740.

Van Breemen, V. L. (1960). Ultrastructure of human muscle. II. Observations on dystrophic striated muscle fibers. Amer. J. Path. *37*, 333–341.

Vanier, T. M. (1960). Dystrophia myotonica in childhood. Brit. Med. J. *2*, 1284–1288.

Walton, J. N. (1955). On the inheritance of muscular dystrophy. Ann. hum. Genet. *20*, 1–38.

Walton, J. N. (1956). The inheritance of muscular dystrophy: further observations. Ann. hum. Genet. *21*, 40–58.

Walton, J. N. (1962). Clinical aspects of human muscular dystrophy. *In* Muscular Dystrophy in Man and Animals. G. H. Bourne and N. Golarz (Eds.). Karger, Basel & New York.

Walton, J. N., and Gardner-Medwin, D. (1969). Progressive muscular dystrophy and the myotonic disorders. *In* Disorders of Voluntary Muscle. J. N. Walton (Ed.). Churchill, London.

Walton, J. N., and Nattrass, F. J. (1954). On the classification, natural history and treatment of the myopathies. Brain *77*, 169–231.

Walton, J. N., and Warrick, C. K. (1954). Osseous changes in myopathy. Brit. J. Radiol. *27*, 1–15.

Wechsler, W., and Hager, H. (1961). Elektronenmikroskopische Untersuchungen bei myotonische Muskeldystrophie. Arch. Psychiat. Nervenkr. *201*, 668–690.

Wohlfahrt, S., and Wohlfahrt, G. (1935). Mikroskopische Untersuchungen an progressiven Muskelatrophien. Acta med. scand. Suppl. *63*, 1–137.

Chapter Five

Collagen Diseases

The various members of the group of conditions called the collagen diseases have important affinities which are still not fully understood in terms of disease pathogenesis. They are diseases of connective tissue ground substance, but their etiology is as yet imperfectly understood. In some of these conditions there is evidence for the important role of auto-immune mechanisms.

The diseases of this group that concern us here are polymyositis, rheumatoid arthritis, polymyalgia rheumatica, systemic lupus erythematosus, systemic sclerosis (scleroderma), rheumatic fever and polyarteritis nodosa. It is also convenient to consider here the condition sarcoidosis.

POLYMYOSITIS

This condition is the most important collagen disease causing disability from involvement of muscle. Formerly it was considered as a variant of the disease dermatomyositis, but now it is recognised that polymyositis is commonly seen without involvement of the skin.

Clinical Findings

The disease occurs mainly in the fifth and sixth decades and is twice as common in females (Pearson 1969). Although the disease is usually seen alone, it also occurs in association with rheumatoid arthritis, scleroderma, disseminated lupus erythematosus and Sjögren's syndrome. There is a special relationship with malignant disease, particularly with carcinomas of the lung, prostate, ovary, uterus, breast and colon.

The clinical presentation of polymyositis is that of muscle weakness of gradual onset, initially affecting the large muscles of the pelvic girdle

94

and followed by involvement of the muscles of the shoulder girdle. Trunk muscles and the distal limb muscles are involved later. In the later stages, the neck muscles, the respiratory muscles and the muscles of the pharynx may be involved. The weakness usually progresses, and in severe cases of long standing, limb contractures may develop. Pain and tenderness of the affected muscles is often present but may not be conspicuous, and insistence on this feature often causes the diagnosis to be missed. Cases do occur without skin involvement, but this accompaniment is common, and in the experience of Pearson (1969), 40 per cent of cases of polymyositis have the characteristic rash of dermatomyositis. This is a dusky erythematous rash over the face which may extend to the forehead, neck, shoulders and arms. Other cases (a further 25 per cent) have minor skin changes ranging from erythema and a desquamating rash to the dermal thickening of scleroderma. The subcutaneous tissue in cases of polymyositis having skin involvement is sometimes oedematous and tender. Raynaud's phenomenon, in which the extremities of the limbs become white or cyanosed following cold or other stimuli, is common (up to 30 per cent of cases). The association of polymyositis with malignant tumours is now undoubted, and this coincidence has been found in one half of cases of polymyositis in males over 40. The tumour is usually a carcinoma; the lung, prostate, ovary, breast and colon have been the sites of the primary tumours. Hodgkin's disease, malignant thymoma and myeloma have also been assoicated with polymyositis.

Clinical Pathology

A neutrophil polymorphonuclear leucocytosis is present, and the erythrocyte sedimentation rate is elevated. The creatine level in the serum and the amount found in the urine are raised. Serum proteins are often altered in that there is an elevation of the α2 and γ globulins. The Rose-Waaler test is often positive. The most valuable tests are of the levels of the serum enzymes, particularly creatine phosphokinase and aldolase, which are always raised in active polymyositis. Levels of glutamic and pyruvic transaminases have also been consistently elevated. These serum enzyme levels are useful in monitoring the progress of the disease, and in judging the effect of treatment.

Neurophysiological Observations

Electromyography consistently shows changes in muscles affected by polymyositis, but the abnormalities are not specific to this disease. They include spontaneous fibrillation potentials, complex polyphasic potentials of small amplitude, and bursts of repetitive potentials of small amplitude. This triad is said to be characteristic of polymyositis (Pearson, 1969).

Pathology

Macroscopically the affected muscles are not obviously abnormal until the later stages of the disease, when there is profound atrophy with fibrous replacement. The histological changes are very striking (Figs. 5–1 to 5–5), and will be described under the following headings: *muscle fibre degeneration, muscle fibre regeneration, inflammatory changes, and fibrotic changes.*

MUSCLE FIBRE DEGENERATION

Muscle fibre degeneration is present in every case, but the amount varies in different cases, in different muscles, and in the same case at different times in the course of the disease (Figs. 5–1 and 5–2). At biopsy in patients dying from the disease in the active phase, all the surviving muscle fibres in the sections may be undergoing degeneration. A degenerating muscle fibre shows hyaline, granular or vacuolar changes in the cytoplasm, which is frequently more eosinophilic than normal. It is characteristic that only a part of the longitudinal extent of a fibre is involved;

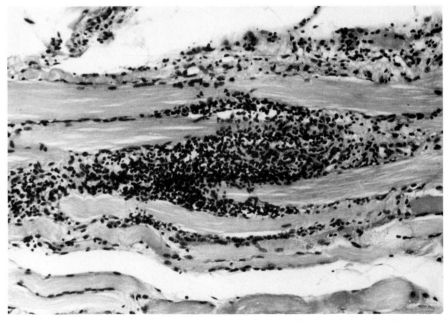

Figure 5–1   Polymyositis. Photomicrograph of longitudinal section of deltoid muscle. The focus of lymphocytes intimately infiltrating between the muscle fibers is characteristic of the disease. The inconspicuous larger macrophages are within degenerating muscle fibers. Note the evidence of regeneration and that sometimes it can be seen that the degeneration only affects part of the muscle fibre. (Haematoxylin and eosin, ×125.)

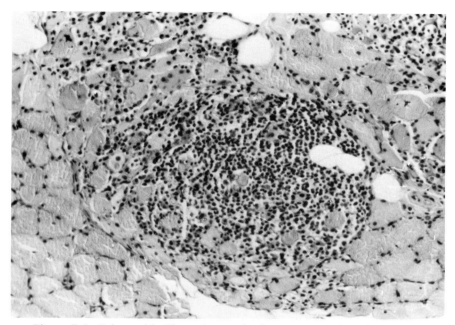

Figure 5–2   Polymyositis. Photomicrograph of transverse section of vastus lateralis muscle. Within the lymphoid focus are many muscle fibres showing degeneration and some fibres showing regeneration. (Haematoxylin and eosin, × 100.)

this partial damage may explain the prominence of regeneration. Complete degeneration of the muscle fibre is followed by phagocytosis, in which the cell is filled with macrophages. The sarcolemmal nuclei become shrunken and pyknotic.

MUSCLE FIBRE REGENERATION

Among the degenerating muscle fibres are others whose appearance is considered to be that of regeneration; these fibres are probably recovering after damage short of total destruction. These so-called regenerating fibres are small, with basophilic cytoplasm and a large vesicular nucleus situated in the centre (Figs. 5–3 and 5–4). Sometimes there are rows of these large central nuclei. In longitudinal sections, the regeneration of a portion of a fibre is sometimes evident as budding from an intact portion of a fibre, or as strands of new growth reaching across a degenerated area to reunite healthy ends of the fibre.

INFLAMMATORY CHANGES

The inflammatory reaction is a very important constituent of the pathology of the disease (Figs. 5–5 to 5–8). It varies considerably in its in-

(Text continued on page 103.)

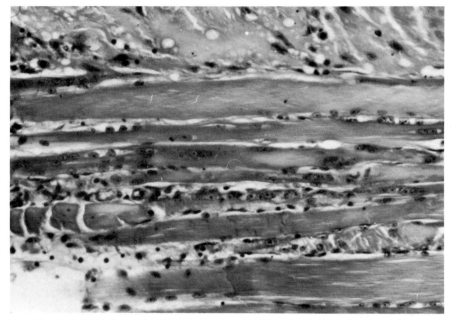

Figure 5-3 Polymyositis. Photomicrograph of longitudinal section from the vastus lateralis muscle of a chronic case. The picture shows regeneration of damaged muscle fibres. Compare with Figures 2-14 and 2-15. (Haematoxylin and eosin, × 185.)

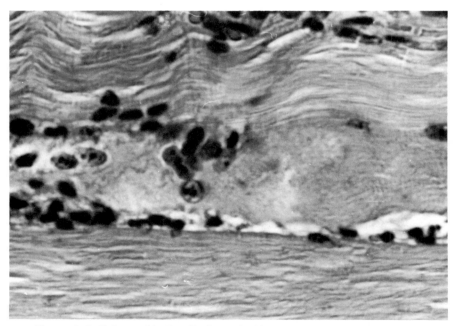

Figure 5-4 Polymyositis. Detail of muscle fibre regeneration seen in Figure 5-3. (Haematoxylin and eosin, × 250.)

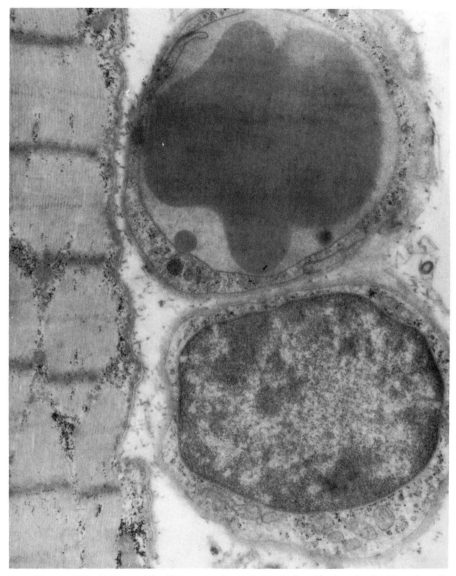

Figure 5-5   Polymyositis. Electron micrograph of ultrathin longitudinal section of muscle. A lymphocyte with increased cytoplasm is seen adjacent to a capillary (2% aqueous uranyl acetate and lead citrate, × 20,000).

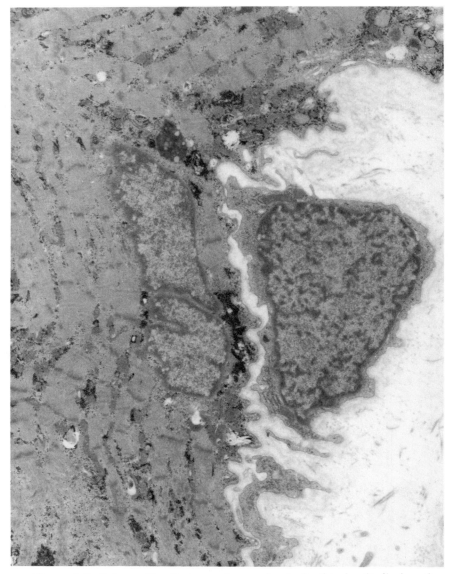

Figure 5–6 Polymyositis. Electron micrograph of ultrathin longitudinal section of muscle. There is an "activated" lymphocyte adjacent to the muscle fibre which shows evidence of degeneration. (2% aqueous uranyl acetate and lead citrate, × 10,000.)

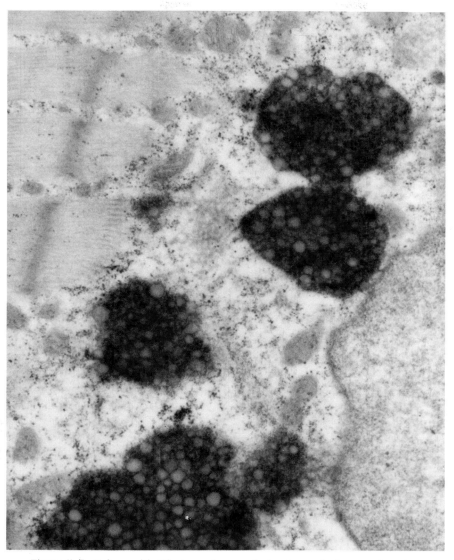

Figure 5–7   Polymyositis. Electron micrograph showing early degenerating changes. The peripheral part of the muscle fibre near the nucleus *(right)* shows degeneration of myofibrils with many lysosomes. (2% aqueous uranyl acetate and lead citrate, × 26,400.)

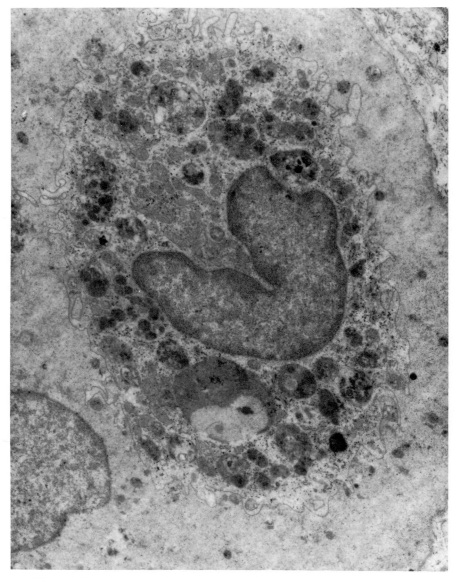

Figure 5-8   Polymyositis. Electron micrograph showing phagocyte within degenerating muscle fibre. (2% aqueous uranyl acetate and lead citrate, × 20,000.)

tensity and extent, and ranges from a few small areas of quiet inflammation to an intense and extensive inflammatory necrosis. In the later stages, when a great deal of muscle has degenerated, there are no inflammatory cells among the fibrous and fatty tissue, but the few surviving muscle fibres are ringed by inflammation. Inflammatory cells are present within the connective tissue septa and around blood vessels, but it is the infiltration among and inside the muscle fibres that is characteristic of polymyositis. The cells forming the inflammatory infiltrate are mainly lymphocytes (Figs. 5–5 and 5–6) or large mononuclears, with some plasma cells. There are many macrophages involved in phagocytosis of the degenerating muscle fibres (Fig. 5–8). Polymorphs and eosinophils are rare. This predominance of lymphocytes and monocytes (the latter may be altered lymphocytes) in the inflammatory infiltrate is of importance in the consideration of the etiology of the disease. It would agree with other evidence that, in this disease, an auto-immune mechanism of damage exists, and the destructive effect is exerted by the sensitisation of lymphocytes.

FIBROTIC CHANGES

More than in many muscle diseases, fibrosis is the prominent sequel to the destruction of muscle fibres. Initially the formation of new vessels and fibroblasts is an important part of the inflammatory reaction; later, extensive fibrosis replaces the lost muscle fibres. Fatty replacement of degenerated muscle also occurs, but is less extensive than in muscle dystrophies.

RHEUMATOID ARTHRITIS

Involvement of muscle is frequently seen in this common disease, and occurs in several ways, which will be considered under the following headings: *neuropathy in R.A.*, *myositis in R.A.*, and *myopathy in R.A.*

Neuropathy in Rheumatoid Arthritis

The existence in rheumatoid arthritis of a peripheral neuropathy and the demonstration of inflammatory foci in peripheral nerve trunks is referred to in the paper by Freund, Steiner, Leichtentritt and Price (1945), and their findings have been confirmed and expanded by, among others, Morrison, Short, Ludwig and Schwab (1947), Hart and Golding (1960) and Haslock, Wright and Harriman (1970). The last-mentioned authors, from their own observations and from an analysis of other recorded cases, consider that there are several types of neural involvement in rheumatoid arthritis. Three forms will be distinguished here.

The first type, which is the commonest, consists of a mild poly-neuropathy affecting predominantly the lower limbs. Examination shows the appropriate sensory disturbance, motor loss and tendon areflexia. Nerve conduction studies give results suggesting slowing of the nerve impulse. The histology of these cases, seen at necropsy and by biopsies on cases, is that of a mixture of axon degeneration and demyelination. The small epineural arteries frequently show subintimal fibrous hyper-plasia, occasionally with obliteration of the lumen. This neuropathy and arteriopathy appears generalised throughout the peripheral nerve trunks, but is more severe distally, and is seen most clearly in the distal parts of the nerves of the lower limbs.

The second type of neuropathy is rarer, and has a more severe clinical form and a bad prognosis. Clinically there is either a widespread polyneuropathy or some form of mononeuritis multiplex. Pathologically there is a severe necrotising arteritis with infarction of nerve trunks, which become severely fibrotic. Axonal degeneration is severe, and there is no obvious preferential loss of myelin, the myelin loss being equal to the axonal loss. This type of neuropathy is very similar to that seen in polyarteritis nodosa; in some of these cases this disease is present in com-bination with rheumatoid arthritis. However, some cases of severe mononeuritis multiplex in rheumatoid arthritis have this localised pa-thology in the nerves, but do not appear to have generalised polyarteritis nodosa.

The third type of nerve lesion in rheumatoid arthritis is that caused to large nerve trunks as they pass near joints deformed by the disease. This is one form of entrapment neuropathy; the commonest example of it is the involvement of the median nerve at the wrist joint.

Myositis in Rheumatoid Arthritis

Steiner, Freund, Leichtentritt and Maun (1946) described their histological findings in the muscles of 14 cases of rheumatoid arthritis which they compared with a large series of normal controls. They dis-covered in all 14 cases, but in none of their controls, a histological abnor-mality which they called "nodular myositis." Several subsequent ob-servers have commented on this finding, which consists of collections of up to 1 mm in diameter of lymphocytes and plasma cells, with occasional mast cells, but without polymorphs or eosinophils. It is important to dis-tinguish these myositic inflammatory collections from the "lymphor-rhages," that have been found in myasthenia (Buzzard, 1905). *Lymphor-rhages* are collections of lymphocytes without an admixture of other inflammatory cells. They are often situated in relation to muscle lym-phatic vessels, and occur commonly in rheumatoid arthritis; however, they are found in many other muscle diseases and are of little diagnostic value. The "nodular myositis" also is of doubtful specificity, and similar collections of chronic inflammatory cells have been seen in skeletal muscle from cases of rheumatic fever, scleroderma and other diseases. A severe polymyositis may be found in rheumatoid arthritis, but in these cases we are probably seeing the coexistence of two related diseases.

In summary, lymphorrhages and myositic nodules occur regularly in the skeletal muscles of patients with rheumatoid arthritis, but are not considered to be specific for this disease. When an extensive myositis is found, this is likely to be the coexistence of the disease polymyositis with rheumatoid arthritis.

Myopathy in Rheumatoid Arthritis

When we have discounted the neurological degenerations and the myositic involvement of skeletal muscle, there remains evidence of some form of myopathy in rheumatoid arthritis. Haslock et al. (1970) described two cases of rheumatoid arthritis in which the muscle fibres showed variation in size, central nuclei, muscle fibre splitting, fibrosis and fatty replacement. These histological changes were suggestive of a muscle dystrophy which, however, was quite unlikely on clinical grounds and from the biochemical investigations. Further study of cases is required for the elucidation of this type of "chronic myopathy" in rheumatoid arthritis. It is tempting to attribute this "myopathic" disorder to forms of therapy, particularly steroid therapy, but this association has been excluded in some of the reported cases.

Another unsolved problem in rheumatoid arthritis is the cause of the severe muscle wasting. Formerly this was attributed to disuse, but experimental methods of producing disuse atrophy by immobilisation indicate that this explanation is unlikely. Muscle atrophy is difficult to produce and to sustain experimentally, even by immobilisation in plaster casts and by tendon detachments. The muscle wasting that is so common even in ambulant patients with rheumatoid arthritis still requires study.

POLYMYALGIA RHEUMATICA

The term polymyalgia rheumatica (Barber, 1957) refers to a condition common in elderly persons who complain of general malaise and myalgic pain and tenderness. There is a mild but definite general body reaction, which often includes pyrexia, and which is evident from a raised erythrocyte sedimentation rate. The condition responds well to treatment with cortisone derivatives (Pauley and Hughes, 1960). There is no obvious arthropathy, and although the muscles would appear from the response to steroid therapy to be involved with a disease process similar to myositis, evidence for this type of disease is lacking. Many muscle biopsies have shown only slight non-specific changes. There is an important association of polymyalgia rheumatica with the disease temporal arteritis. In this latter disease the tunica media of certain extracranial arteries, notably the superficial temporal artery, is involved by a granulomatous giant-celled inflammatory reaction that often causes thrombosis. Temporal arteritis can lead to blindness, and any failure of vision in a case of polymyalgia rheumatica requires investigation. Massive cortisone therapy can preserve the eyesight in these cases.

SYSTEMIC LUPUS ERYTHEMATOSUS

The name *systemic lupus erythematosus* is now preferred to that of *disseminated lupus erythematosus* for the generalised form of this disease; when the condition appears restricted to the skin, the term *discoid lupus erythematosus* is used. The unity of these two forms of the disease has been clear since the LE-cell test (Hargreaves, Richmond and Morton, 1948) brought precision to the diagnosis of the disease. This test has also demonstrated that the condition is much commoner than was hitherto recognised.

The systemic form of lupus erythematosus may affect most organs and tissues. The organs most commonly affected are the heart, lungs, liver, spleen, kidneys and lymph nodes. The tissues most commonly affected are skin, blood vessels, synovial tissue and skeletal muscle. The common pathological changes in these various locations are destruction of tissue, a chronic inflammatory reaction, fibrinoid change seen in connective tissue or in the walls of blood vessels, and the presence of haematoxylin-stained bodies. Less commonly, the necrosis of tissue takes the form of miliary granulomata. A good description of the pathological changes in various organs and tissues in the generalised disease is that of Cruikshank (1966).

Involvement of skeletal muscle in *systemic lupus erythematosus* is well known, and takes the form of muscle tenderness usually affecting the upper arms and thighs. Weakness may be present, but the main disability is caused by pain. Subcutaneous calcification may occur. In patients with severe muscle involvement, the serum enzyme levels are elevated, sometimes to a marked degree (Dubois, 1966). The electromyogram shows changes similar to those seen in polymyositis.

The pathological findings in muscle from cases of *systemic lupus erythematosus* have been described by Klemperer, Pollack and Baehr (1941), reporting on necropsy cases, and by Erbslöh and Baedeker (1962), examining necropsies and muscle biopsies. The findings have been those of partial or complete degeneration of muscle fibres and an inflammatory reaction consisting of lymphocytes, histocytes and plasma cells. Fibrinoid change was found in vessel walls, and occasionally there was endarteritis with occlusion. Haematoxylin-staining bodies and miliary granulomata do not appear to have been observed in skeletal muscle.

Many authors have made the point (Cruikshank, 1952) that the changes seen in muscle in lupus erythematosus cannot be satisfactorily distinguished from those found in rheumatoid arthritis, polyarteritis nodosa, scleroderma and polymyositis. In the extensive examination permitted at necropsy, these different diseases usually can be distinguished, and in the interpretation of muscle biopsies the clinical picture should be taken into account. A simultaneous skin biopsy may also be helpful.

Reports have appeared (Pearson and Yamazaki, 1958) of a vacuolar myopathy (Hughes, Esiri, Oxbury and Whitty, 1971) that is caused by chloroquine therapy. This drug has been used extensively in the treatment of lupus erythematosus, and there is a strong suspicion that, in many of the cases of vacuolar myopathy seen in this disease, the cause has been chloroquin therapy.

SYSTEMIC SCLEROSIS

The term scleroderma was originally used for a disorder confined to the skin, but it is now known that this disease process can affect a wide range of body tissues. One convention uses *morphea* for cases of scleroderma in which the disease is localised to skin and *systemic sclerosis* to describe cases with widespread disease. Scleroderma has been considered a disease of collagen since collagen diseases were separated as a group (Klemperer, Pollack and Baehr, 1942). Systemic sclerosis is found more often in females than in males, and begins in the age range of 30 to 50 years (Sackner, 1966). The condition affects the skin, heart, lungs, alimentary tract, kidneys, bones and joints, and muscles.

The involvement of muscles has long been recognised (Robert, 1890), but clinically it is rare to have more than slight weakness, cramp-like pains, and tenderness. With severe skin involvement, the underlying subcutaneous tissues and muscles may be contracted.

The pathological changes found in the muscles are those of a myositis not very different from that seen in polymyositis. There is usually more arteritis and commonly a thickening, often gross, of the interstitial connective tissue septa in the muscles.

RHEUMATIC FEVER

Acute rheumatic fever, formerly a common disease of childhood, has now become rare in Britain and America, and at the same time, the cases that do occur have less severe manifestations (Markowitz and Kuttner, 1965). The disease appears to be closely related to a throat infection by the group A beta-haemolytic streptococcus, and an antibody against streptolysin O is found in the serum of patients from about one week after the throat infection. It is not yet clear whether the disease is a hypersensitivity reaction to the group A streptococcus or an auto-immune disorder.

The chief clinical manifestations of rheumatic fever are heart disease, joint disease, chorea, rheumatic subcutaneous nodules and erythema marginatum. A myositis of voluntary muscle is usually present, but this feature is often overshadowed by the more serious cardiac manifestations.

The characteristic pathology seen in the heart, joints and subcutaneous nodules is the Aschoff body (Aschoff, 1904), which is a perivascular accumulation of large macrophages around a centre of fibrinoid necrosis. This structure has been seen in the connective tissues of muscles (Shaw, 1929), but the findings in the bundles of muscle fibres are of a non-specific myositis (Adams, Denny-Brown and Pearson, 1967). Further observations on the pathological changes in skeletal muscle in rheumatic fever are required. For the present we must consider the muscle changes as a non-specific myositis made up of collections of chronic inflammatory cells.

POLYARTERITIS NODOSA

Rokitansky, and later Kussmaul and Maier (1866), made the first descriptions of the pathological changes in the clinical entity now called polyarteritis nodosa or periarteritis nodosa. The condition is not rare; it occurs at any age, but has a peak incidence in the fifth and sixth decades, and affects men twice as commonly as women.

It presents with protean manifestations because the causative arteritis is generalised throughout most of the organs and tissues of the body. In order of frequency, cardiac, renal, muscular, cutaneous, alimentary, neurological and respiratory involvement may occur. No specific laboratory test has been found for the disease. There is a moderate neutrophil leucocytosis, often with an eosinophilia. The E.S.R. is raised, often markedly, and the renal damage can sometimes be demonstrated by finding red cells in the urine. A recent development has been the demonstration of Australia antigen in the blood of some cases (Gocke, Hsu, Morgan, Bombardieri, Lockshin and Christian, 1970).

Muscle involvement in polyarteritis nodosa is common, and a muscle biopsy is frequently undertaken to confirm the disease. A survey of the results of biopsy, made by Maxeiner, MacDonald and Kirklin (1952), found 35 per cent positive biopsies in cases believed to be polyarteritis nodosa. The incidence of positive findings increased when tender nodules could be palpated at the site of the biopsy in cases in which symptoms had been present for over six months.

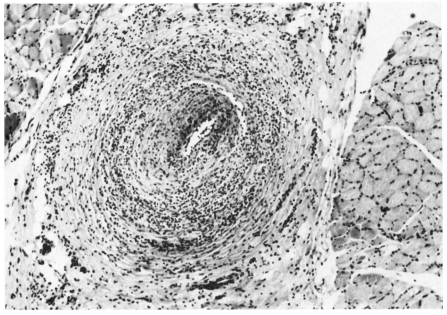

Figure 5–9 Polyarteritis nodosa. Photomicrograph of deltoid muscle showing a large muscle artery. There is a panarteritis affecting all the muscle wall and causing severe narrowing of the lumen. (Haematoxylin and eosin, × 25.)

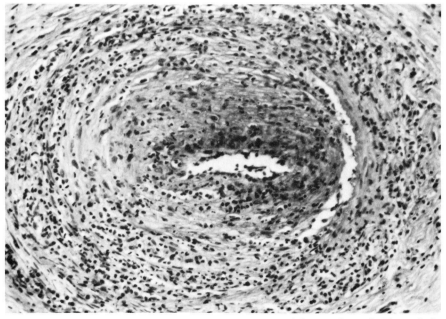

Figure 5–10 Polyarteritis nodosa. High power view of the vessel seen in Figure 5–9. Many of the inflammatory cells are polymorphonuclear neutrophil leucocytes. (Haematoxylin and eosin, × 50.)

The characteristic pathology is an arteritis of small to medium sized arteries affecting a short segment of a vessel or a small arc of a vessel wall (Figs. 5-9 and 5-10). The nodose form with small aneurysms, which figured predominantly in the early reports, is uncommon. Thrombosis of affected arteries is common. The cellular infiltration characteristically affects the media and adventitia, or the intima, media and adventitia, and consists in the early stages of polymorphs and eosinophils (Fig. 5-10). Later, macrophages are common. The arterial wall shows hyaline fibrinoid necrosis with positive staining for fibrin. Sometimes small granulomata are present; these may contain "foreign body" giant cells.

SARCOIDOSIS

Sarcoidosis is the name now generally used to embrace all the manifestations of a generalised systemic disease due to an abnormal state of tissue reactivity to some stimulus, which is often the tubercle bacillus. Scadding (1967) prefers to define the disease in pathological terms, as "a disease characterised by the presence in all of several affected organs or tissues of epithelioid cell tubercles, without caseation though some fibrinoid necrosis may be present at the centres of a few tubercles, proceeding either to resolution or to conversion of the epithelioid cell tubercles into avascular hyaline fibrous tissue." The organs most frequently affected in sarcoidosis are the lymph nodes, lungs, liver, spleen, skin, eyes, small bones of the hands and feet, and the salivary glands. In common with all organs and tissues, muscles can be affected either as a subclinical myopathy in a case of sarcoidosis or, more rarely, as a myositis presenting with a clinical picture of muscle weakness. Both forms of muscle involvement have clinical importance.

Subclinical Myositis in Sarcoidosis

It is now clear from observations made on muscle biopsies that, despite the absence of symptoms and signs, infiltration of skeletal muscle by sarcoid granulomata is frequently present in the early active phase of sarcoidosis, especially in those cases of acute onset with fever, arthralgia or erythema nodosum. The pathological findings have been described by Wallace, Lattes, Malia and Ragan (1958); Myers, Gottlieb, Mattman, Eckley and Chason (1952); and by Powell (1953). At this early stage there are small sarcoid granulomata situated perivascularly in the connective tissue septa and sometimes within muscle fibres. A moderate lymphocytic infiltration is frequently present. Atrophied muscle fibres may be present and are probably due to denervation from sarcoid involvement of spinal nerve roots or peripheral nerve trunks.

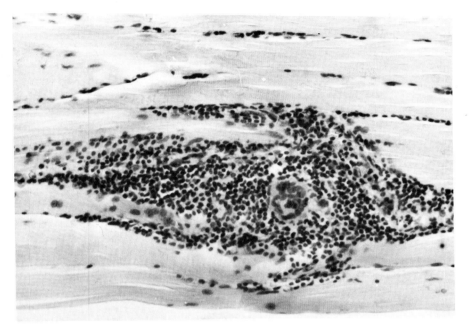

Figure 5–11   Sarcoidosis. Photomicrograph of longitudinal section of deltoid muscle. There is destruction of muscle fibres by a small sarcoid granuloma. (Haematoxylin and eosin, ×60.)

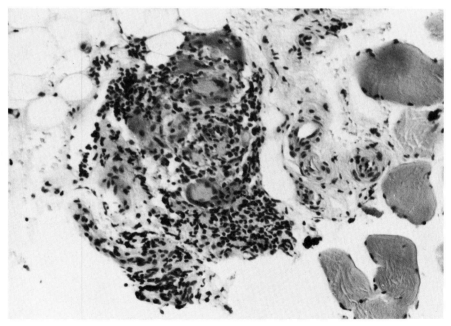

Figure 5–12   Sarcoidosis. A sarcoid granuloma is seen in the interstitial tissue of a transverse section. (Haematoxylin and eosin, ×60.)

Clinical Myositis in Sarcoidosis

Sometimes in sarcoidosis the muscle involvement is sufficient to cause weakness and wasting of muscle groups; in these cases the presence of palpable nodules in the affected muscles is likely. These cases are of two types. The most usual form is a polymyositis accompanying sarcoidosis of other organs or tissues. The papers of Weinberger (1933), Powell (1953), Coërs, Durand, Malmendier and Wittek (1956) and of Crompton and MacDermott (1961) refer to cases of this type. Much more rarely, as in the cases reported by Snorasson (1947), Warburg (1958) and Brun (1961), the myositis dominates the clinical picture and there is no indication of systemic sarcoidosis elsewhere.

Diagnosis by Muscle Biopsy

Because of this common involvement of skeletal muscle, muscle biopsy is an important diagnostic measure in a case of sarcoidosis (Figs. 5–11 and 5–12). The myositis appears to be widespread, and the large proximal limb muscles, which are accessible to biopsy, are usually involved. Before biopsy, these muscles should be carefully palpated in a search for small tender nodules, where positive histological findings are much more likely.

References

Adams, R. D., Denny-Brown, D., and Pearson, C. M. (1967). Diseases of Muscle. 2nd ed. Hoeber, New York.

Aschoff, K. A. L. (1904). Zur Myocarditisfrage. Verh. Dtsch. Ges. Pathol. *8*, 46–51.

Barber, H. S. (1957). Myalgic syndrome with constitutional effects. Ann. Rheum. Dis. *16*, 230–237.

Brun, A. (1961). Chronic polymyositis on the basis of sarcoidosis. Acta psychiat. Scand. *36*, 515–523.

Buzzard, E. F. (1905). The clinical history and post-mortem examination of five cases of myasthenia gravis. Brain *27*, 438–483.

Coërs, C., Durand, J., Malmendier, G., and Wittek, M. (1956). Un cas de sarcoïdose avec insuffisance rénale et entreprise musculaire généralisée. Acta clin. belg. *11*, 348–364.

Crompton, M. R., and Macdermott, V. (1961). Sarcoidosis associated with progressive muscular wasting and weakness. Brain *84*, 62–74.

Cruikshank, B. (1952). Focal lesions in skeletal muscles and peripheral nerves in rheumatoid arthritis and other conditions. J. Path. Bact. *64*, 21–32.

Cruikshank, B. (1966). The basic pattern of tissue damage and pathology of SLE. Chapter 2 *in* Lupus Erythematosus. E. L. Dubois (Ed.). McGraw-Hill, New York.

Dubois, E. L. (1966). The Clinical Picture of Systemic Lupus Erythematosus. Chapter 5 *in* Lupus Erythematosus. E. L. Dubois (Ed.). McGraw-Hill, New York.

Erbslöh, F., and Baedeker, W. D. (1962). Lupus Myopathy. Dtsch. Med. Wochenschr. *87*, 2464–2470.

Freund, H. A., Steiner, G., Leichtentritt, B., and Price, A. E. (1945). Nodular polymyositis in rheumatoid arthritis. Science *101*, 202–203.

Gocke, D. J., Hsu, K., Morgan, C., Bombardieri, S., Lockshin, M., and Christian, C. L. (1970). Association between polyarteritis and Australia antigen. Lancet *2*, 1149–1153.

Hargreaves, M. M., Richmond, H., and Morton, R. (1948). Presentation of two bone marrow elements: the "Tart" cell and "L.E." cell. Proc. Staff Meet. Mayo Clin. *23*, 25–28.

Hart, F. D., and Golding, J. R. (1960). Rheumatoid neuropathy. Brit. Med. J. *1*, 1594–1600.

Haslock, D. I., Wright, V., and Harriman, D. G. F. (1970). Neuromuscular disorders in rheumatoid arthritis. Quart. J. Med. *39*, 335–358.

Hughes, J. T., Esiri, M., Oxbury, J. M., and Whitty, C. W. M. (1971). Chloroquine Myopathy. Quart. J. Med. *40*, 85–93.

Klemperer, P., Pollack, A. D., and Baehr, G. (1941). Pathology of disseminated lupus erythematosus. Arch. Path. (Chicago) *32*, 569–631.

Klemperer, P., Pollack, A. D., and Baehr, G. (1942). Diffuse collagen disease; acute disseminated lupus erythematosus and diffuse scleroderma. J.A.M.A. *119*, 331–332.

Kussmaul, A., and Maier, R. (1866). Ueber eine bisher nicht beschriebene eigenthumliche Artemenerkrankung, die mit Morbus Brightii und rapid fortschreitender allgemeiner Muskellahmung einhergeht. Dtsch. Arch. klin. Med. *1*, 486.

Markowitz, M., and Kuttner, A. G. (1965). Rheumatic Fever. W. B. Saunders Company, Philadelphia.

Maxeiner, S. R., MacDonald, J. R., and Kirklin, J. W. (1952). Muscle biopsy in the diagnosis of periarteritis nodosa. Surg. Clin. N. Amer. *32*, 1225–1233.

Morrison, L. R., Short, C. L., Ludwig, A. O., and Schwab, R. S. (1947). Neuromuscular system in rheumatoid arthritis; electromyographic and histologic observations. Amer. J. Med. Sci. *214*, 33–49.

Myers, G. B., Gottleib, A. M., Mattman, P. E., Eckley, G. M., and Chason, J. L. (1952). Joint and skeletal muscle manifestations in sarcoidosis. Amer. J. Med. *12*, 161–169.

Pauley, J. W., and Hughes, J. P. (1960). Giant-cell arteritis, or arteritis of the aged. Brit. Med. J. *2*, 1562–1567.

Pearson, C. M. (1969) Polymyositis and related disorders. *In* Disorders of Voluntary Muscle. J. N. Walton (Ed.). Churchill, London.

Pearson, C. M., and Yamazaki, J. N. (1958). Vacuolar myopathy in systemic lupus erythematosus. Amer. J. Clin. Path. *29*, 455–463.

Powell, L. W. (1953). Sarcoidosis of skeletal muscle — report of 6 cases and review of literature. Amer. J. Clin. Path. *23*, 881–889.

Robert, G. (1890). Des myopathies dans la sclerodermie. Thèse de Paris.

Sackner, M. A. (1966). Scleroderma. Grune & Stratton, New York.

Scadding, J. G. (1967). Sarcoidosis. Eyre & Spottiswoode, London.

Shaw, A. F. B. (1929). Topography and pathogenesis of lesions in rheumatic fever. Arch. Dis. Child. *4*, 155–164.

Snorrason, E. (1947). Myositis fibrosa progressiva in patient with lymphogranulomatosis benigna Boeck. Nord Med. *36*, 2424–2425.

Steiner, G., Freund, H. A., Leichtentritt, B., and Maun, M. E. (1946). Lesions of skeletal muscles in rheumatoid arthritis; nodular polymyositis. Amer. J. Path. *22*, 103–145.

Wallace, S. L., Lattes, R., Malia, J. P., and Ragan, C. (1958). Muscle involvement in Boeck's sarcoid. Ann. Intern. Med. *48*, 497–511.

Warburg, M. (1958). A case of symmetrical muscular contracture due to sarcoidosis. J. Neuropath. Exp. Neurol. *14*, 313–315.

Weinberger, M. (1933). Uber eine Chronisch verlaufere Polymyositis mit Ausgang in progressive Muskelatrophie. Wien. med. Wochenschr. *83*, 100; 137; 162.

Chapter Six

Microbial Diseases

A large variety of microbial agents have been incriminated in the causation of certain muscle infections, but with the exception of Bornholm disease, caused by the Coxsackie virus group, and certain parasitic infestations, none of these diseases are at all common. The subject will be considered under the following headings: *viruses, bacteria,* and *parasites.*

VIRUSES

Virus infections of muscle are uncommon; indeed, virus infections of all mesodermal structures are rare compared with the abundance of examples of infection of ectodermally derived tissues. The main exception to this generalisation is the Coxsackie group of viruses, which readily infect the muscles of laboratory animals and which cause the clinical condition of Bornholm disease. The development of modern techniques of virus indentification in human tissues may in the future demonstrate many more viruses involving human muscle; two examples of possible pathogens for which complete evidence is lacking will be mentioned here. Norris, Dramov, Calder and Johnson (1969) described two cases of myositis occurring during an attack of herpes zoster. In each case electron microscopical studies of excised muscle revealed virus-like particles in the sarcoplasm of muscle fibres. Middleton, Alexander and Szymanski (1970) reported from Toronto a series of 26 children with bilateral lower limb myalgia lasting one to five days and associated with an upper respiratory tract infection and the recovery of influenza virus from nasopharyngeal secretions. Twenty-two of the cases occurred in an epidemic in March and April of 1969 from influenza B virus, and three in the month of January 1970 from A2 Hong Kong influenza virus. Another case from influenza B virus occurred in April 1970.

114

Bornholm Disease

This condition, which is also termed epidemic myalgia, pleurodynia and Devil's grip, was first described in the second half of the nineteenth century. An excellent monograph on the disease is that of Sylvest (1934).

The first descriptions of epidemics are credited to Finsen, who in 1856 and 1863 described cases in Iceland. Homann in 1972 and Daae in 1874 described cases in Norway. Dabney in 1888 described a large epidemic in Virginia, U.S.A. More recent reports are those of Finn, Weller and Morgan (1949) and of Warin, Davies, Sanders and Vizoso (1953). The common name for the disease comes from the Danish island of Bornholm where in 1930 a Danish doctor (Sylvest, 1934) was holiday-making with his family, who contracted the disease in an epidemic present on the island.

Epidemics of Bornholm disease occur in summer and early autumn, attacking most often children between 5 and 15 years, and affecting males and females equally. The incubation period is from two to four days, when pain on inspiration or movement begins in certain muscles, notably the muscles of the hypogastrium and epigastrium but also the muscles of the chest, back, loins and shoulders. The affected muscles are painful, aching and tender. Palpation of the tender areas may reveal localised swelling or rigid firm areas. Because of pain, breathing may be shallow or hurried, and hiccup may be present if the diaphragm is involved. There is usually a febrile reaction, with a neutrophil polymorphonuclear leucocytosis and eosinophilia in the blood. The acute illness lasts from one to seven (usually four) days, and complete recovery occurs. Rarely, however, there are relapses, and second attacks can occur. Of the severe complications (meningitis, pneumonia, pleurisy, otitis media), only orchitis is common, and the pathology of the testis in Bornholm disease appears to be similar to that of mumps orchitis. Since the first association of the group B Coxsackie virus with this disease (Curnen, Shaw and Melnick, 1949), this virus has been consistently recovered from the faeces of cases. Attempts at isolation of the virus from C.S.F., blood, and throat washings have usually failed.

No fatal cases of Bornholm disease have been described, and there are no descriptions of necropsies of cases. Findings in muscle biopsies from two cases were reported by Lépine, Desse and Sautter (1952), who described muscle fibre necrosis with phagocytes and a mononuclear inflammatory infiltration. The pathology of the experimental infection in newborn mice is well known, and is used as a diagnostic test of the isolation of the virus (Dalldorf and Melnick, 1965).

Virus-like Particles in Polymyositis

Until recently, most virus diseases were considered to be acute infections. In this light, Bornholm disease would be a typical example—a highly infectious, epidemic disease, giving rise to a short illness presumably due to the invasion of the skeletal muscles by the Coxsackie virus. This narrow concept of viral disease has now been enlarged by recent discoveries of the persistence of virus in human tissues and of chronic diseases caused by viruses actively present in tissues over long periods. This new thinking prompts a search for viruses in cases of chronic polymyositis. Already a few interesting reports have appeared.

Chou (1968) found, by electron microscopy, virus-like particles in the nuclei and cytoplasm of muscle fibres from three muscle biopsies spanning a time interval of 18 months in a case of polymyositis. He interpreted the morphological appearance of the virus as a myxovirus. Chou and Gutmann (1970) and Mastaglia and Walton (1970) have described virus-like particles similar to picorna-virus in the muscle fibre cytoplasm of cases of polymyositis. These reports are extremely interesting but as yet it is not possible to say whether these virus agents are directly responsible for the disease or whether they invade muscle of persons having a susceptibility for viral infections which are secondary to the principal disease. The illustrations of virus particles (Figs. 6–1 and 6–2) accompanying this chapter are from one of two such cases of polymyositis studied in the author's laboratory.

BACTERIA

Only in special circumstances do certain bacteria thrive in skeletal muscle. Of these predisposing states, mention should be made of trauma, pressure sores and the spread of infection from neighbouring septic foci. The gas-gangrene group of organisms cause a particular form of septic myositis; rarely, skeletal muscles are involved by tuberculosis or syphilis. The invasion of muscle fibres by the leprosy bacillus has an important place in the understanding of the disease.

Trauma

Crushing injuries or penetrating wounds, particularly when contaminated by foreign material, are common sites of bacterial infections which, before the availability of chemotherapy and antibiotics, were dreaded complications of open wounds. The streptococcus and staphylococcus were most often the cause, but at the present time it is the resistance of an organism to specific therapy which determines its dominance in wound infection. Organisms thus brought into prominence are *Proteus vulgaris* and *Pseudomonas aeruginosa*.

Pressure Sores

Decubitus ulceration from the effect of pressure causes septic areas which may be extensive and frequently involve muscle. A variety of organisms may be present.

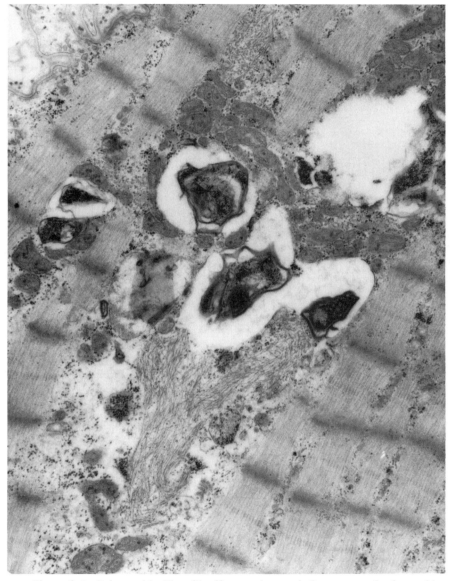

Figure 6–1   Polymyositis. Virus-like filaments in muscle from a case of polymyositis. The electron micrograph shows part of the edge of a muscle fibre cut longitudinally. There is degeneration of myofibrils with the formation of "myelin" figures. Large numbers of filaments are present in the space created by the degeneration of a myofibril. (2% aqueous uranyl acetate and lead citrate, × 20,000.)

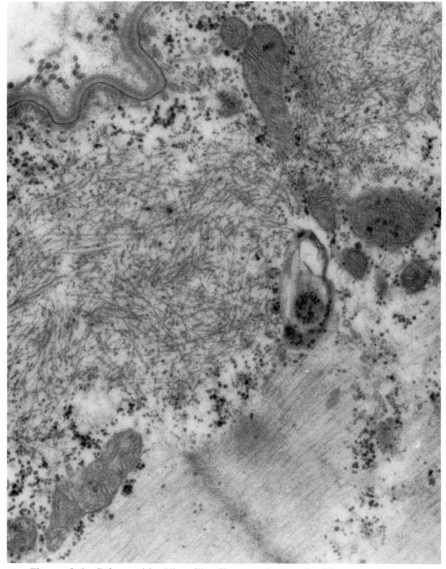

Figure 6–2   Polymyositis. Virus-like filaments in muscle. Electron micrograph at higher magnification showing the detail of the filaments seen in Figure 6–1. (2% aqueous uranyl acetate and lead citrate, × 40,000.)

Neighbouring Septic Foci

Bacterial myositis and abscess formation may occur as a spread from septic foci, the commonest example being pyogenic osteomyelitis.

Gas Gangrene

This is a special type of bacterial myositis that has great importance in certain surgical conditions. It is most evident as an infection of severe traumatic incidents, either civilian injuries or battle wounds. The predisposing factor is an extensive muscle injury which is contaminated with soil or other foreign material containing the spores of the causative organism *(Clostridium welchii, C. oedematiens)*. These organisms do not attack healthy living tissues, but can grow in dead tissue under anaerobic conditions (Figs. 6–3 to 6–5). The muscle fibres are decomposed rapidly by the bacterial multiplication. The striations are lost, and the staining of the sarcoplasm and nuclei becomes indistinct. The mechanism of the progression of the gangrenous process depends on the elaboration by the bacteria of toxins and digestive enzymes. A more specialised but related condition is tetanus caused by the toxin produced by *Clostridium tetani*.

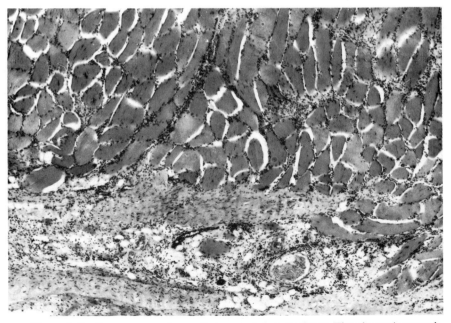

Figure 6–3   Gas gangrene. Lower limb amputation specimen. The photomicrograph shows the inflammatory oedema in the muscle at the advancing edge of the septic infarction. (Haematoxylin and eosin, × 20.)

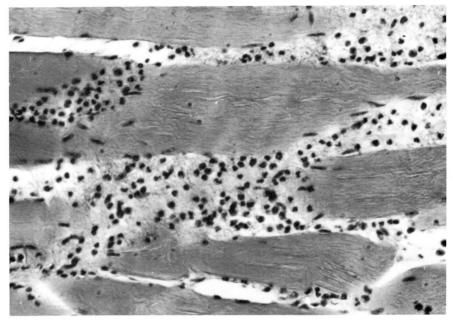

Figure 6–4   Gas gangrene. Detail of myositis. Note the oedema and the acute inflammatory exudate between individual muscle fibres. (Haematoxylin and eosin, × 60.)

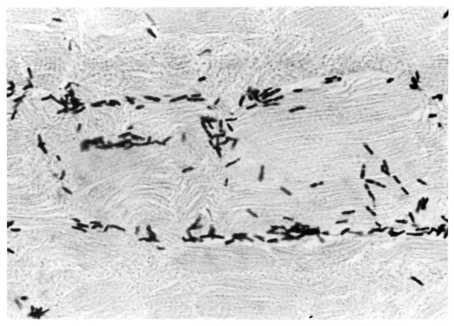

Figure 6–5   Gas gangrene. Detail of anaerobic spore-bearing bacilli which spread mainly between the muscle fibres. (Gram's stain, × 180.)

Tuberculosis

This is a rare infection of muscle, except by spread into the paravertebral muscles from tuberculous osteomyelitis of the spine (Figs. 6–6 and 6–7). The resultant psoas abscess is a very characteristic accompaniment to Pott's disease of the spine.

Syphilis

Gumma can occur in various muscles, but the incidence of this complication of syphilis is now rare. Even more uncommon is a diffuse myositis caused by syphilis. Most references to this condition are in the medical literature of the nineteenth century.

Leprosy

It has recently been shown, first in the experimental animal (Esiri, Weddell and Rees, 1972) and subsequently in biopsies from human cases

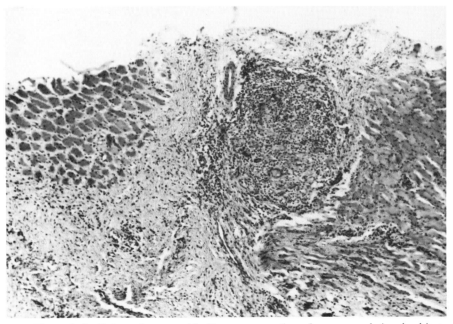

Figure 6–6 Tuberculous myositis. Transverse section of psoas muscle involved in a chronic granulomatous infection by tuberculosis. Note the fibrosis, the chronic inflammatory reaction, and the nodule of tuberculous inflammation. (Haematoxylin and eosin, × 40.)

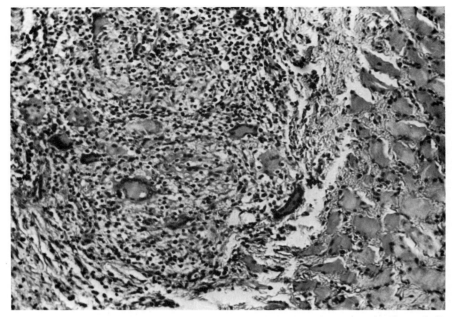

Figure 6–7 Tuberculous myositis. Detail of tuberculous focus seen in Figure 6–6. (Haematoxylin and eosin, × 85.)

(Pearson, Rees and Weddell, 1970), that striated muscle fibres are colonised by *Mycobacterium leprae* at an early stage of the disease (Figs. 6–8 and 6–9). The bacteria thrive within the sarcoplasm without at first causing much damage to the muscle fibre, which thus plays an important part in the multiplication of the bacteria. Smooth muscle is also invaded, and in the human disease the involvement of the dartos muscle under the skin is probably of great importance.

PARASITES

Among the parasitic infestations that affect skeletal muscle, only trichiniasis and cysticercosis are common human diseases. Toxoplasmosis also involves muscle, but causes trivial disability in this location compared with its manifestations in the central nervous system.

Trichiniasis

This widespread disease is caused by a small whipworm called the *Trichinella spiralis*. There are three main stages in the life cycle of the parasite (Fig. 6–10). The *adult form* is a worm located in the small intestine of

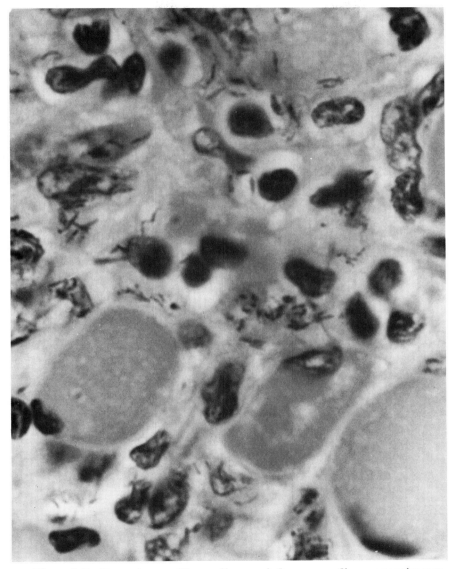

Figure 6–8   Human leprosy. Biopsy of leg muscle from a case of lepromatous leprosy. Colonies of lepra bacilli are present within degenerating muscle fibres, as described by Pearson, Rees and Weddell, 1970. (Fite-Faraco modification of Ziehl-Neelsen technique. Approx. × 400.) (Photomicrograph kindly provided by Professor A. G. M. Weddell.)

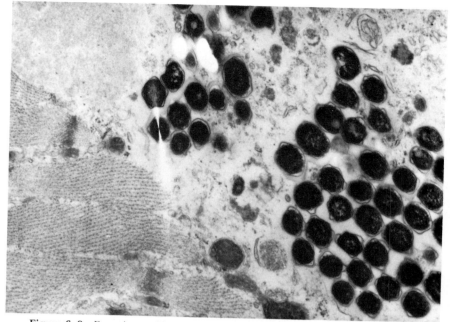

Figure 6–9 Experimental leprosy in a mouse. Colony of Mycobacterium leprae in a foot-pad striated muscle fibre. (Uranyl acetate and lead citrate, × approx. 20,000.) (Electron micrograph kindly provided by Dr. M. M. Esiri.)

the host. The male adult worm is about 1.5 mm long and the female about 3.5 mm long. The *embryonal form*, which hatches out from eggs in the uterus of the worm and passes into the small intestine of the host, measures about 100 μ in length. The *larval form* is predominantly found in muscles where the trichinellae consist of oval capsules about 1 mm long, made up of a host connective tissue reaction, and containing one to four coiled worms having a blunt or rounded head end and a slender pointed tail.

This parasite can infect most animals (except birds), but in nature and in animal husbandry the pig and the rat are the most important hosts. Animals are infected by consuming the offal and flesh of other infected animals; lack of hygiene in the feeding of pigs and lack of rat control are causes of the disease in herds of swine. Man is infected by eating inadequately cooked pork containing cysts of the *T. spiralis*, which can survive moderate heating.

Once the cysts are consumed, they hatch out in the small intestine into male and female adult worms which become mature in about a week. The eggs laid by the female hatch out in the uterus of the parasite and then are discharged into the lumen of the small bowel. They penetrate into the small bowel mucosa and thence migrate via lymphatics and veins into the blood stream, from which they invade the skeletal muscles.

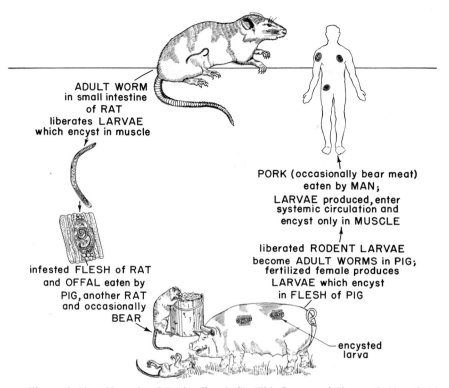

Figure 6–10   Life cycle of *Trichinella spiralis*. (This figure and Figures 6–11 to 6–14 are reproduced by permission from Ash, J. E., and Spitz, S. (1945). Pathology of Tropical Disease. W. B. Saunders Company, Philadelphia.)

CLINICAL FINDINGS

Three phases of the clinical disease of trichiniasis can be recognised (Manson-Bahr, 1966).

1. THE STAGE OF INVASION.   This stage begins 7 to 14 days after infection and may be manifest as an enteritis, which can be very severe, with abdominal pains, violent diarrhea and vomiting.

2. THE STAGE OF THE MIGRATION OF LARVAE.   This stage may not cause clinical symptoms, but frequently there is a high fever with an encephalopathy.

3. THE STAGE OF MYOSITIS.   The third stage gradually succeeds the second, usually about four weeks after infection. There is a high fever which may be intermittent or remittent. There are frequently skin eruptions with pruritus and often oedema, particularly of the face and notably affecting the eyelids. The myositis affects many muscles but particularly the diaphragm, intercostals, eye muscles, neck muscles and the large limb muscles near their tendinous insertions. The affected muscles are weak, painful, swollen and tender, particularly with movement,

which is restrained. Eosinophilia is common and may account for 50 per cent of a total leucocyte count of 20,000 to 35,000. Recovery in a few weeks is the rule, but weakness may persist for months. There can be considerable mortality (from to 1 to 20 per cent), depending on the severity of the infection.

PATHOLOGY OF THE MUSCLE

The trichinellae may be seen in muscle biopsies and in necropsied cases. In the examination of animal carcasses, muscle is searched by the digestion of large quantities of muscle in artificial gastric juice. Teased portions of fresh unfixed muscle are used to demonstrate motility in the living larvae. The gross appearance of muscle infested by trichinellae can be characteristic. The muscles are pale, with greyish or whitish streaks according to the stage of the disease during which fibrosis is succeeded by calcification. The encysted larva consists of a short, curved worm or a long, spirally coiled form, according to the stage of growth (Figs. 6–11 and 6–12). Initially the worm occupies part of a muscle fibre, but in later stages most of the fibre has degenerated and the larva occupies all of the cross sectional area of the fibre. The parasite is sur-

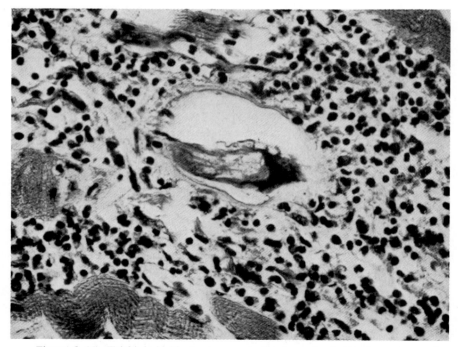

Figure 6–11   Trichiniasis. Photomicrograph showing a developing larva among degenerating muscle fibres. The surrounding exudate consists chiefly of plasma cells and lymphocytes.

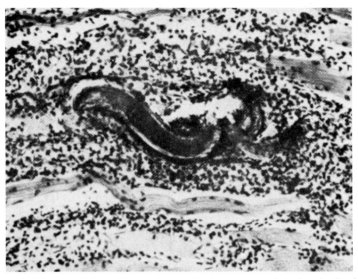

Figure 6–12   Trichiniasis. Photomicrograph showing muscle in longitudinal section. The developing larva is beginning to elongate into a spiral form. Note the intense myositis and oedema.

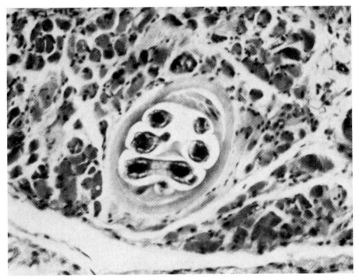

Figure 6–13   Trichiniasis. Photomicrograph showing a fully developed encysted larva with a hyalin capsule. The myositis has subsided but calcification of the cyst has not yet begun.

rounded by a prominent inflammatory exudate composed of polymorphs and eosinophils (Figs. 6–11 and 6–12). The nature of the
enclosing fibrous capsule depends also on the stage of the disease. Initially the capsule is composed of a thin fibrous layer but later it becomes
thick (Fig. 6–13) and, on the death of the parasite, will calcify. Regeneration activity is prominent in muscle affected with trichiniasis. When seen
in a late stage with a lymphocytic inflammatory reaction, a diagnosis of
polymyositis may be wrongly made.

Cysticercosis

This disease results from the presence in man of the larval form of
the pork tape worm *Taenia solium*. Normally, man harbours the adult

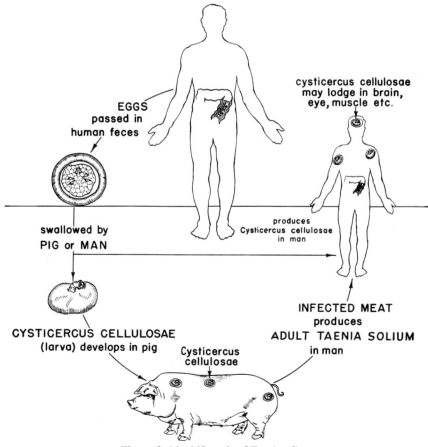

Figure 6–14   Life cycle of *Taenia solium*.

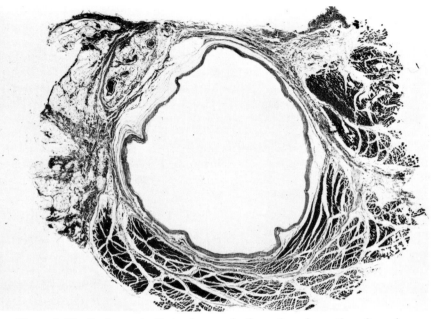

Figure 6–15   Cysticercosis. Photomicrograph of a section of a portion of muscle containing a cysticercus removed for biopsy. The parasite has formed a thin-walled cyst surrounded by a fibrous capsule derived from the host. (Haematoxylin and eosin, × 2.)

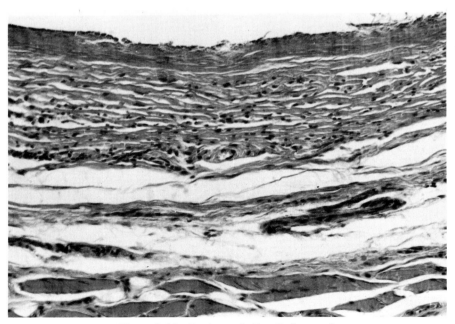

Figure 6–16   Cysticercosis. Detail of cyst wall.

worm as an intestinal parasite, the intermediate host of the larval form being the pig (Fig. 6–14). In cysticercosis, man is infected by the accidental ingestion of ova from human faeces, or possibly by proglotides containing ova moving upward into the stomach by reverse peristalsis. The *ova* hatch out in the stomach and upper small intestine, and the larvae migrate throughout the body, invading the muscle and subcutaneous tissue and most body organs; notably the brain and eyes. The *larvae* can remain alive for many years and cause most disability when they die, liberating a toxic product to which the body reacts. *Cysticercosis* is common in India and in most eastern countries, and is seen in Britain and in the United States as epilepsy presenting several years after residence in these countries.

CLINICAL FINDINGS

There may be a previous history of an intestinal tapeworm but this story is not often obtained. The stage of invasion of the larvae may cause some generalised malaise and pyrexia, but often passes unregarded. The more characteristic finding is the appearance of subcutaneous swellings in crops, commonly affecting the lips, tongue, masseter muscles, neck, trunk and groin. These nodules are firm and slightly tender, and range from 0.5 to 2 cm in diameter. In addition there may be more generalised muscle tenderness and weakness. Eosinophilic leucocytosis is usually present. The diagnosis of the disease as a myositis is rather uncommon. More often the appearance of epilepsy eventually leads to the diagnosis of cerebral involvement long after the initial infection. X-rays of limb and trunk muscles may show calcified cysts, but only several years after infection.

PATHOLOGICAL FINDINGS

Excision of a subcutaneous or intramuscular nodule, or the biopsy of a tender muscle, may show the parasite in the form of a cyst surrounded by a fibrous capsule derived from the host tissues (Figs. 6–15 and 6–16). The live parasite has only a thin surrounding capsule, but after its death dense fibrosis and calcification will occur. Fresh specimens should be teased out of the containing capsule when the thin translucent surrounding membrane with a central "milk spot" is characteristic of the species.

References

Chou, S. M. (1968). Myxovirus-like structures and accompanying nuclear changes in chronic polymyositis. Arch. Path. (Chicago) *86*, 649–658.

Chou, S. M., and Gutmann, L. (1970). Picornavirus-like crystals in subacute polymyositis. Neurology (Minneap.) *20*, 205–213.

Curnen, E. C., Shaw, E. W., and Melnick, J. L. (1949). Disease resembling non-paralytic poliomyelitis associated with a virus pathogenic for infant mice. J.A.M.A. *141*, 894–901.

Dalldorf, G., and Melnick, J. L. (1965). Coxsackie viruses. Chapter 19 *in* Viral and Rickettsial Infections of Man. 4th ed. F. L. Horsfall and I. Tamm. (Eds.). Lippincott, Philadelphia.

Esiri, M. M., Weddell, A. G. M., and Rees, R. J. W. (1972). Infection of murine striated muscle with *Mycobacterium leprae*: a study by light and electron microscopy. J. Path. Bact. *106*, 73–80.

Finn, J. J., Weller, T. H., and Morgan, H. R. (1949). Epidemic pleurodynia; clinical and etiological studies based on 114 cases. Arch. Intern. Med. *83*, 305–321.

Lépine, P., Desse, G., and Sautter, V. (1952). Biopsies musculaires examen histologique et isolement du virus coxsackie chez l'homme atteint de myalgie épidémique (maladie de Bornholm). Bull. Acad. Natl. Méd. (Paris) *136*, 66–69.

Manson-Bahr, P. G. (1966). *Manson's Tropical Diseases.* Baillière, Tindall and Cassell, London.

Mastaglia, F. L., and Walton, J. N. (1970). Coxsackie virus-like particles in skeletal muscle from a case of polymyositis. J. neurol. Sci. *11*, 593–599.

Middleton, P. J., Alexander, R. M., and Szymanski, M. T. (1970). Severe myositis during recovery from influenza. Lancet *2*, 533–535.

Norris, F. H., Dramov, B., Calder, C. D., and Johnson, S. G. (1969). Virus-like particles in myositis accompanying herpes zoster. Arch. Neurol *21*, 25–31.

Pearson, J. M. H., Rees. R. J. W., and Weddell, A. G. M. (1970). *Mycobacterium leprae* in the striated muscle of patients with leprosy. Lepr. Rev. *41*, 155–166.

Sylvest, E. (1934). *Epidemic Myalgia.* Oxford University Press, Oxford.

Warin, J. F., Davies, J. B. M., Sanders, F. K., and Vizoso, A. D. (1953). Oxford epidemic of Bornholm disease, 1951. Brit. Med. J. *1*, 1345–1351.

Chapter Seven

Toxic Myopathies

The term myopathy, as used in this book, means any pathological state of muscle, and therefore, to indicate a particular disease state, it should be qualified by an adjective. Using this convention, the term *toxic myopathy* is readily understood. Many different toxic substances have been reported to cause myopathies, although the actual number of cases seen is much smaller than the number of cases of denervating, dystrophic and myositic diseases. Toxins can be exogenous or endogenous, but most instances of toxic myopathy are due to exogenous toxins, which can be subdivided into drugs and poisons. The most important toxic myopathy is probably alcoholic myopathy. The condition known as Haff disease will be included in this chapter, although as yet there is no proof that a poison is the cause of this myopathy.

MEDICAL DRUGS CAUSING MYOPATHY

The myopathies produced by steroids and by antimalarial drugs will be described in detail. Mention will be made of the myotoxicity of the following drugs: vincristine, succinylcholine, bretylium tosylate and the sulphonamides.

Steroid Myopathy

A variety of steroids have been responsible for myopathy, and the following drugs have been incriminated: *cortisone* (Perkoff, Silber, Tyler, Cartwright and Wintrobe, 1959); *prednisone* (Harman, 1959); *triamcinolone* (Williams, 1959; Strandberg, 1962); *fludrocortisone* (MacLean and Schurr, 1959); and *dexamethasone* (Golding, Murray, Pearce and Thompson, 1961). ACTH therapy has also given rise to myopathy (Yates, 1963).

132

CLINICAL FEATURES

There is no exact relationship between the duration of the steroid treatment or the amount of steroids given and the appearance of the myopathy. Possibly individual susceptibility to steroids is important. Usually, however, a dose of 15 to 20 mg per day has caused myopathy in three to six months (Yates, 1970). The patient tires easily and cannot ascend stairs or perform simple tasks requiring the muscles of the shoulder girdle. There are accompanying features of cortisone intoxication, such as a hirsute appearance, striae, moonface and buffalo-hump adiposity. Clinical examination discovers weakness of the large proximal muscles and of the trunk.

CLINICAL PATHOLOGY

Elevation of serum enzymes has not been shown to occur in steroid myopathy, if one excludes the cases of muscle disease (in particular, polymyositis) which are being treated with steroids. Electromyography has sometimes given abnormal results (Yates, 1970).

HISTOPATHOLOGY

Reports of the histological changes in steroid myopathy differ, but all agree that the changes seen by light microscopy are slight. Perkoff *et al.* (1959) described the pathological changes in muscle as minimal. Golding *et al.* (1961) said that conventional histological examination revealed only minor changes. The four cases examined by motor-point muscle biopsy by Haslock, Wright and Harriman (1970) showed no light microscope changes either in the muscle or in its innervation.

ULTRASTRUCTURAL CHANGES IN STEROID MYOPATHY

Many observations on the ultrastructural changes of muscles from patients receiving steroids have been made (Figs. 7–1 to 7–4), in addition to studies on cases of steroid myopathy. The results have been variable and conflicting, and it is difficult as yet to ascribe any of the ultrastructural changes to steroids. What has been described is "myofilament loss," dilatation of the sarcoplasmic reticulum (Figs. 7–1 and 7–2), excess glycogen (Figs. 7–3 and 7–4), and excess of intracellular fat. There are more observations from studies on experimental animals, but these cannot be applied to the human situation without some caution.

ETIOLOGY OF STEROID MYOPATHY

While there seems no doubt of the reality of steroid myopathy as a clinical state, the paucity of morphological changes in the affected

(Text continued on page 138.)

Figures **7–1** to **7–4**   Cortisone myopathy. Case of ulcerative colitis treated for long periods with cortisone, and developing marked weakness of the muscles of the shoulder and pelvic girdles. Improvement followed cessation of cortisone therapy. Biopsy of the deltoid muscle showed only minor light microscopic changes.

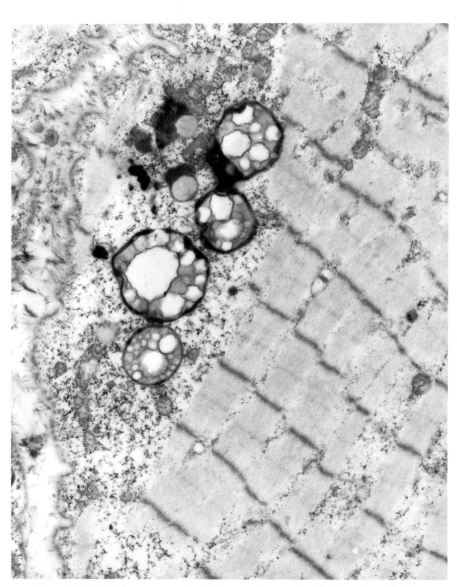

Figure 7–1   Cortisone myopathy. Electron micrograph of edge of muscle fibre cut longitudinally. Note the lipid bodies and the dilated triads of the sarcoplasmic reticulum. (2% aqueous uranyl acetate and lead citrate, × 12,000.)

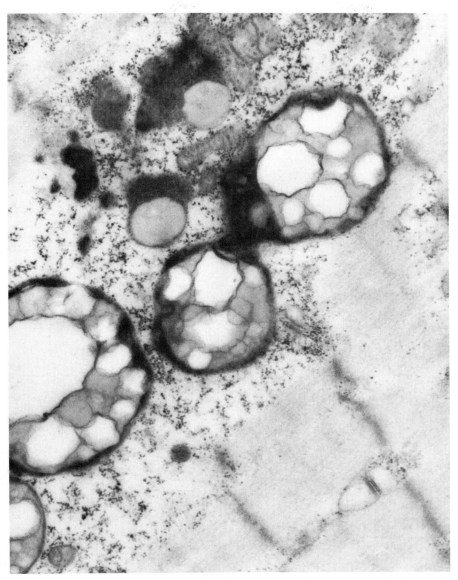

Figure 7–2   Cortisone myopathy. Detail at higher magnification of part of picture of Figure 7–1. (2% aqueous uranyl acetate and lead citrate, × 26,500.)

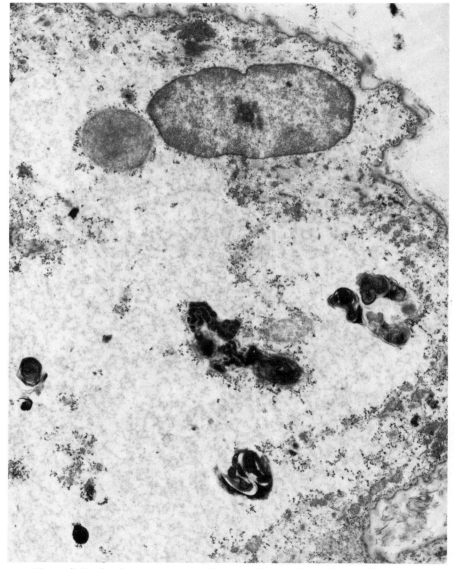

Figure 7–3 Cortisone myopathy. Electron micrograph of the peripheral part of a muscle fibre affected by advanced degeneration. All the elements of contractile protein have been lost. There is an excess of glycogen with many lysosome-like structures. (2% aqueous acetate and lead citrate, × 6000.)

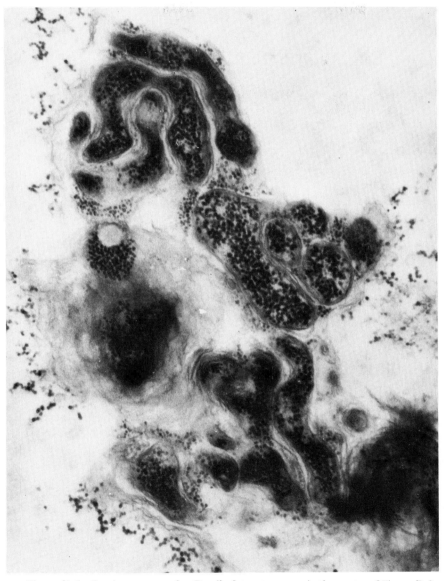

Figure 7–4   Cortisone myopathy. Detail of structure seen in the centre of Figure 7–3. There are concentric membranes enclosing glycogen granules. Compare with the myelin figures of Figure 7–8. (2% aqueous uranyl acetate and lead citrate, × 40,000.)

muscles is puzzling, and there is no obvious lead to understanding the nature of the muscle defect.

Chloroquine Myopathy

The effect of chloroquine in producing a myopathy in experimental animals was described by Nelson and Fitzhugh (1948) several years before the first cases of chloroquine myopathy in human patients were reported. Chloroquine given as the sulphate or phosphate was originally introduced as an antimalarial drug, but has since been recognised as a valuable therapeutic in rheumatoid arthritis and lupus erythematosus. It is also used occasionally in skin photosensitivity, glomerulonephritis and sarcoidosis. Cases of chloroquine myopathy have been reported by Whisnant, Espinosa, Kierland and Lambert (1963); Loftus (1963); Begg and Simpson (1964); Garcin, Rondot and Fardeau (1964); Blom and Lundberg (1965); Blomberg (1965); Renier (1965); Milligen and Suerth (1966); Ebringer and Colville (1967); Hicklin (1968); Panahi, Braun, Guiraudon and Delbarre (1968); Chapman and Ewen (1969); and by Hughes, Esiri, Oxbury and Whitty (1971).

CLINICAL FEATURES

Myopathy has followed the use of chloroquine only when the drug has been administered in a high and continuous dosage for periods of a year or more. The absorption of chloroquine is rapid and complete, but excretion of the drug is very slow, and consequently there is a cumulative effect. A course of high dosage (e.g., 300 to 500 mg per day for one or two years) leads, perhaps inevitably, to a toxic concentration that will cause myopathy. The lower dosages used in malarial prophylaxis (e.g., 400 mg per week) have not been shown to cause myopathy.

The weakness is most apparent in the limbs and affects mainly the proximal muscles, although the trunk muscles are often simultaneously involved. In severe cases, all the muscles — even those supplied by cranial nerves — may be affected. It is now clear (Hughes *et al.*, 1971) that the heart is simultaneously affected, and death from cardiomyopathy has been seen. Some of the clinical reports suggest that there is neural involvement; this has been demonstrated in experimental work. In most of the human cases the myopathy predominates and is the cause of the weakness. The serum enzymes may be moderately elevated. Electromyography has sometimes shown abnormalities.

HISTOPATHOLOGY

The light microscopic appearance of the muscle in chloroquine myopathy is striking. Sections show a gross disorder of the muscle fibres,

(*Text continued on page 142.*)

Figures **7–5** to **7–8**   Chloroquine myopathy. Case 2 of Hughes *et al.* (1971). Prolonged treatment with chloroquine was given for sarcoidosis.

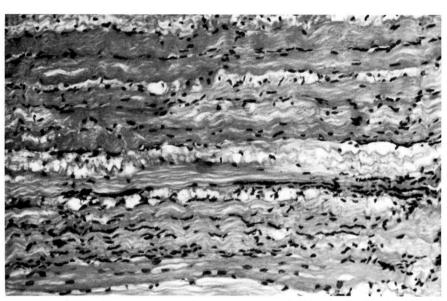

Figure 7–5   Chloroquine myopathy. Photomicrograph of longitudinal section of right vastus lateralis muscle. About half the muscle fibres are degenerating. (Haematoxylin and eosin, × 110.)

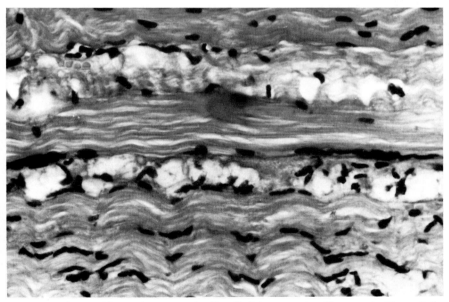

Figure 7–6   Chloroquine myopathy. Detail of degenerating fibre seen in Figure 7–5. Note the vacuolar degeneration affecting some of the muscle fibres. (Haematoxylin and eosin, × 250.)

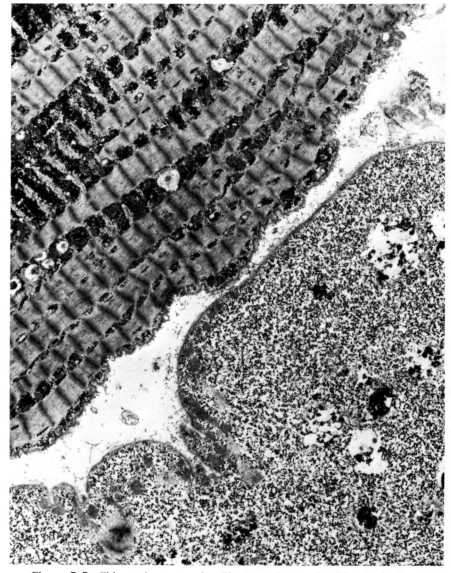

Figure 7–7   Chloroquine myopathy. Electron micrograph of longitudinal section showing two adjacent muscle fibres. Above and to the left is an agranular (type II) fibre which shows very little abnormality. The fibre below and on the right shows severe degeneration. (2% aqueous uranyl acetate and lead citrate, × 6000.)

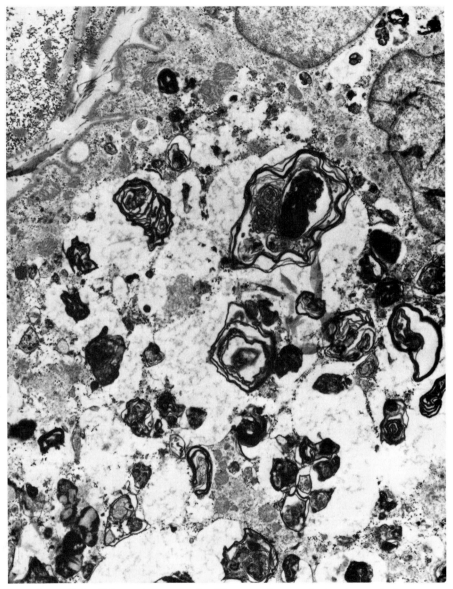

Figure 7-8 Chloroquine myopathy. Electron micrograph showing part of a degenerating muscle fibre. There are countless "myelin figures" formed by concentric lamellae of electron-dense membranes. Some are compound structures enclosing smaller figures. (2% aqueous uranyl acetate and lead citrate, × 8000.)

approximately one half of which are affected by a vacuolar degeneration (Figs. 7–5 and 7–6). The affected muscle fibres are swollen and the muscle sarcoplasm is fragmented into homogenous masses. In these fibres the sarcolemmal nuclei are numerous and are often situated in the centre of the fibre. The vacuoles are conspicuous, and when they are numerous and occupy the whole of the fibre they give rise to a vesicular appearance. This vesicular appearance is distinct from the changes in McArdle's syndrome in which the vacuoles are situated peripherally. The severe degeneration of the muscle is not accompanied by an inflammation reaction, and there are no particular changes in the interstitial connective tissue or in the muscle vessels.

Histochemical examination of the muscle has shown that the process attacks preferentially the granular (type I) muscle fibres. The interpretation of the histochemical reactions is not easy, because the degenerating fibres are rich in all the enzymes commonly found in muscle.

ULTRASTRUCTURE OF CHLOROQUINE MYOPATHY

The electron microscope has shown, as has histochemical examination, that there are two populations of muscle fibres: those of one population undergo severe degeneration, whereas those of the second group are normal or show only minor changes (Fig. 7–7). The fibres not undergoing degeneration appear to be non-granular (type II) fibres.

The architecture of the degenerating muscle fibres shows severe disruption (Fig. 7–8). The band structure is almost totally destroyed and there are only a few surviving fragments of sarcomeres. The main content of the muscle fibre is a mass of glycogen granules, among which are electron-dense bodies, some of which resemble the lysosomes seen in many muscle diseases. The majority of the electron-dense bodies are not the usual lysosomes but structures called "myelin figures" (Fig. 7–8). These have concentric lamellae of thin, continuous electron-dense membranes. Sometimes two or more myelin figures are enclosed by other concentric membranes to form compound structures. Mitochondrial degenerative changes are prominent and appear to be the first stage in the formation of the myelin figures.

The sarcolemmal nuclei are displaced to the centre and appear increased in number. The sarcolemma appears infolded The sarcoplasmic reticulum and the transverse tubular system has been destroyed in the degenerating type I fibres but appears normal in the surviving type II fibres.

ETIOLOGY OF CHLOROQUINE MYOPATHY

The ultrastructural changes, the preferential involvement of the granular (type I) fibres, and the involvement of the heart can all be explained by a direct toxic action of chloroquine on mitochondria. Mitochondrial degeneration has been consistently demonstrated in cases of chloroquine myopathy and in experimental chloroquine intoxication. The other important feature is the stabilising effect of chloroquine on the membranes of lysosomes (Weissmann, 1969); this effect may explain the formation of the striking myelin figures.

Vincristine Myopathy

The alkaloid vincristine sulphate obtained from the periwinkle *Vinca rosea* is used in the treatment of neoplasms, and in particular in the treatment of acute leukaemia in children. Reports on its use (e.g., Martin and Compston, 1963) describe a neurological complication that is considered to be a toxic polyneuropathy. Whether myopathy is also present requires further investigation of patients on this drug. In experiments with rats (Slotwiner, Song and Anderson, 1966) a profound myopathy can be produced by vincristine, which in rats causes no neurological degeneration. The myopathy in the experimental animals is characterised by progressive degeneration of the muscle fibres, which contain interfibrillar spheromembraneous bodies up to 3 μ in diameter; these are thought to be a degeneration product formed from sarcoplasmic reticulum and mitochondria.

Succinylcholine Myopathy

Injections of succinylcholine during halothane anaesthesia (Airaksinen and Tammisto, 1966) have been incriminated in the causation of a myopathy.

Bretylium Tosylate Myopathy

This condition is referred to by Gardner-Medwin and Walton (1969).

Sulphonamide Myopathy

Lisander (1970) described a 30-year-old man who on three occasions developed muscle pain resulting from courses of sulphametin. Allergic reactions had occurred in this individual from penicillin, streptomycin and horse serum. It is possible that the myopathy also was caused by a sensitivity to sulphonamides, and so was not a true form of toxicity.

POISONS CAUSING MYOPATHY

Of the many poisons known to cause myopathy, only alcohol and the postulated poison of the mysterious Haff disease have caused more than a few cases. These two conditions will be described in detail; other myotoxic poisons will be mentioned more briefly.

Alcoholic Myopathy

Although the neuropathy that may complicate chronic alcoholism is well known, the several varieties of myopathy that may also occur have only recently attracted attention. Reference to a myopathic state can actually be found in the earlier descriptions of the peripheral neuropathy of alcoholism (Siemerling, 1889; Gudden, 1896), but recognition of the distinctive features of alcoholic myopathy dates from the papers of Hed and his co-authors (Hed, Larsson and Wahlgren, 1955; Hed, Lundmark, Wahlgren and Orell, 1962) in Scandinavia. Many reports have followed with accounts of the clinical state (Perkoff, Diaso, Bleisch and Klinkerfuss, 1967; Lafair and Myerson, 1968), and of the light and electron microscope findings in the muscle (Klinkerfuss, Bleische, Diaso and Perkoff, 1967; Lynch, 1969; Kahn and Meyer, 1970).

Alcoholic myopathy occurs as an acute myopathy, as a chronic myopathic state, and as a subclinical state detectable only by clinical and biochemical investigations in cases of chronic alcoholism. The different types may only represent differences in exposure to alcohol, and the chronic myopathic state may be ushered in by an attack of acute myopathy.

ACUTE ALCOHOLIC MYOPATHY

This is the most dramatic form of the condition. It invariably occurs in a chronic alcoholic and is precipitated by a recent prolonged bout of heavy drinking. The muscles particularly affected are the proximal limb muscles and the muscles of the abdominal wall, and in these very painful cramps are experienced. The muscles are extremely tender, and there may be swelling and oedema of the overlying subcutaneous tissues. Myoglobinuria is often present and may lead to death from acute renal failure (Valaitis, Pilz, Oliner and Chomet, 1960). Recovery from the acute myopathy may take place within a few weeks if the patient abstains from alcohol.

CHRONIC ALCOHOLIC MYOPATHY

The chronic myopathic state may follow an episode of acute alcoholic myopathy or it may arise insidiously. It appears as a progressive weakness accompanied by pain and tenderness, and affects mainly the proximal limb muscles. This chronic myopathic state may last several months, but recovery is possible if reasonable temperance is maintained.

Subclinical Alcoholic Myopathy

Subclinical cases have been found during surveys of chronic alcoholics. Examination of large series of chronic alcoholics discovers these subclinical cases who have muscle weakness and tenderness, and positive clinical and biochemical tests. This subclinical state is also reversible if abstention from alcohol can be maintained.

CLINICAL PATHOLOGY

In the acute myopathy there is severe muscle necrosis causing marked elevation of serum enzyme levels and often myoglobinuria. In the chronic myopathy, and to a lesser extent in the subclinical myopathy, increased urinary excretion of creatine and creatinine and moderate elevation of serum enzyme levels have been found. The ischaemic exercise test, in which the forearm is exercised with an inflated pressure cuff on the arm, is often positive; i.e., the procedure causes severe cramp-like pain, and following the exercise there is no rise in the blood lactate estimated in a venous blood sample. Electromyography has often been normal but has sometimes shown changes of denervation.

HISTOPATHOLOGY

In *acute alcoholic myopathy* the histological appearances depend on the stage of the disease and whether the muscle examined is severely or moderately affected. The muscle fibres show necrosis, which may be hyaline, granular or vacuolar (Fig. 7–9). The necrosis may affect only part of the fibre, and the sarcolemmal sheath may be intact. This partial damage to the muscle fibre may explain the prominence of features of regeneration. These features include the presence of small muscle fibres with basophilic cytoplasm and rows of large vesicular nuclei with large nucleoli. The other feature frequently present is an excess of fat as droplets within the muscle fibres and as fatty infiltration of the endomysium between individual muscle fibres.

In *chronic alcoholic myopathy* the changes seen in histological sections are much less evident. There is an increase in the connective tissue of the perimysium and endomysium, and in these locations there is more neutral fat than normal. An increase in fat can be demonstrated within the muscle fibres.

ULTRASTRUCTURAL CHANGES

The electron microscopic appearances of alcoholic myopathy have been frequently studied (Figs. 7–10 and 7–11). In acute alcoholic myop-

Figures **7–9** to **7–11**   Alcoholic myopathy. Case of chronic alcoholism developing painful weakness of proximal limb muscles.

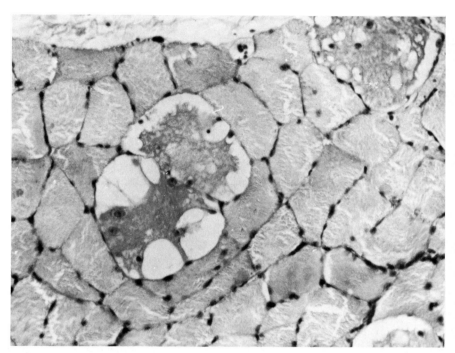

Figure 7–9   Alcoholic myopathy. Photomicrograph of transverse section of triceps muscle. A vacuolar degeneration affects a few of the muscle fibres. (Haematoxylin and eosin, × 250.)

athy the degenerating muscle fibre shows a moderate increase in volume, with excessive cytoplasm separating the myofibrils. The myofibrils are abnormal in that there is irregularity of the in-step arrangement of the bands, which are also variable in width. Many myofilaments are lost, and those remaining are disoriented. The sarcoplasmic reticulum and the T-system are only slightly dilated.

In *chronic alcoholic myopathy* many large lipid droplets can be seen throughout some of the muscle fibres whose band structures are abnormal, particularly with respect to the I band. Mitochondria are decreased in number, and often contain dense bodies in their matrices. There are irregular spaces between myofibrils, and in these can be found amorphous electron-dense material amidst many glycogen granules. Presumably in the *subclinical form of alcoholic myopathy*, which can be recognised by a positive exercise-ischaemia test and by the presence of raised serum enzyme levels, similar but less marked changes will be found to those

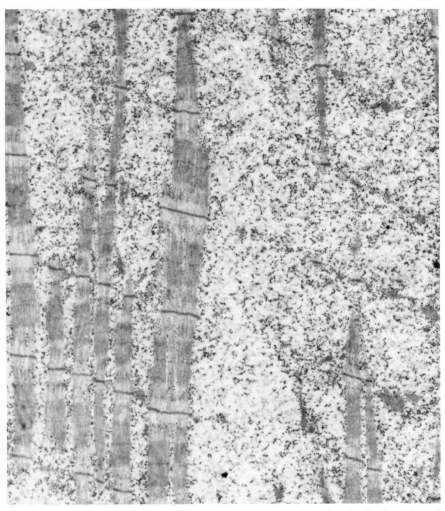

Figure 7–10   Alcoholic myopathy. Electron micrograph of longitudinal section of muscle fibre. The myofibrils are attenuated by loss of myofilaments. There is a conspicuous increase in glycogen. (2% aqueous uranyl acetate and lead citrate, × 8000.)

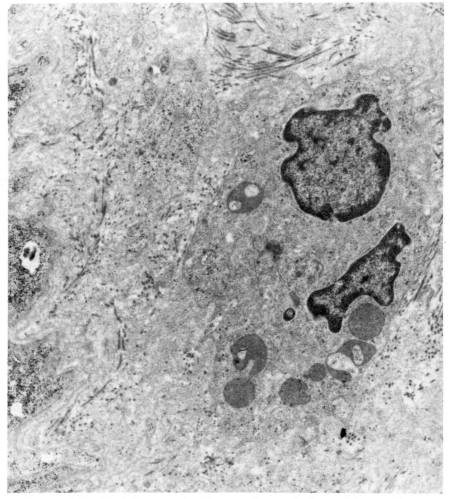

Figure 7-11   Alcoholic myopathy. Electron micrograph of part of degenerating muscle fibre containing phagocytes. (2% aqueous uranyl acetate and lead citrate, × 11,000.)

described here under chronic alcoholic myopathy. As yet there are no reports of any specific ultrastructural changes in the muscle fibres in any of these forms of alcoholic myopathy.

ETIOLOGY OF ALCOHOLIC MYOPATHY

Several theories have been proposed to explain the myopathy of chronic alcoholism. The most informative link that has been demonstrated is the similarity of alcoholic myopathy to the congenital metabolic disease known as McArdle's syndrome (Perkoff *et al.*, 1967). In both conditions the exercise-ischaemia test fails to elevate the blood lactate. Phosphorylase activity is low in alcoholic myopathy, although, unlike in McArdle's syndrome, glycogen is not present in the muscle in excessive amounts. Another theory is that a toxic effect of alcohol on the muscle cell membrane wall or on mitochondria may cause intracellular oedema. The sarcoplasmic reticulum and the T-system have not been shown to be markedly changed, and so abnormal shift of tissue fluid appears not to be a factor in causing the myopathy.

The studies of Fewings, Hanna, Walsh and Whelan (1966) indicate a vasoconstrictor effect of alcohol on the vessel walls of muscular arteries, and possibly an ischaemic mechanism causes the muscle necrosis. Further observations are required on this interesting effect of alcohol on muscle.

Haff Disease

In the second half of 1924 and in the first half of 1925 a mysterious myopathy occurred in epidemic form around the shores of the Koenigsberg Haff in East Prussia. Because of its chief manifestation it has been called *paroxysmal myoglobinuria*, but the term Haff disease is more widely used. A second major epidemic occurred in the same region in late 1932 and early 1933, and a smaller epidemic was seen in 1940. An epidemic of cases of a similar nature occurred around the shores of Lake Onega in Russia in 1934 and in Sweden early in 1942 around the shores of Lake Yinsen near Mariestad in the province of Skaraborg (Berlin, 1948).

CLINICAL PICTURE

The clinical presentation of a case is striking. The patient has always consumed a meal of fish, usually the day preceding the onset of the illness. The patient becomes acutely ill, with intense pain beginning in the legs and back and rapidly spreading to all the muscles of the body except those of the head. The pain and tenderness in the muscles are excruciating, and the slightest movement is resisted. The first passage of urine after the onset of the illness is usually blackish brown in colour, and sometimes red. Acute renal failure may occur and may cause death. Apart from the renal complications, which are due to capillary obstruction of glomerular filtration by myoglobin, the disease appears restricted to muscle; there is no mental deterioration and no peripheral neuropathy. There is no arthropathy, except that all movements are resisted because of the pain. The patients are afebrile, and there is only a moderate neutrophil leucocytosis. There is no anaemia.

PATHOLOGY OF THE MUSCLE

The histological appearance of the muscle in Haff disease has not been extensively studied except for the early German descriptions of the first epidemic. The histochemistry and the electromicroscopy of the muscle in this disease would be of great interest, but its capricious appearance has so far prevented this type of study.

CAUSE OF HAFF DISEASE

This remains a complete mystery, and the only lead is that the patients have consumed fish. Sea birds, cats and foxes have also suffered from the condition. Earlier an explanation based on an industrial effluent containing sulphites was favoured, but the later epidemic in Sweden occurred on the shores of a lake which had no industrial development. No specific bacteria or virus has been isolated from the fish or from the human cases. An analogy has been drawn between Haff disease and Chastek disease, the latter being a myopathy seen among the captive silver foxes on the silver fox farms in North America. Chastek's disease can be produced by a vitamin B_1 deficiency, and it is said that the fishes fed to the foxes may contain a substance which inactivates vitamin B_1.

Carbon Monoxide Myopathy

Several reports have appeared (Mautner, 1955; Loughridge, Leader and Bowen, 1958; Jackson, Bunker and Elder, 1959) suggesting that carbon monoxide poisoning can cause a myopathy. These cases arise from suicidal or accidental poisoning, and often the patient has lain for some time in coma. Anoxia both general and local, due to pressure from the abnormal posture while the patient is unconscious, is thought to be the main factor in these cases.

Snake Venoms

The active principle of some snake venoms is an anticoagulant (e.g., that of the Indian cobra). Others—particularly those of the snakes belonging to the family *Hydrophidae* — are strongly myotoxic. These snakes are tropical marine snakes of which about 500 species exist, distributed widely in the islands of the Pacific Ocean and around the coasts of Asia, North Australia and the tropical parts of the Americas. The beaded seasnake, *Enhydrina schistosa*, has given rise to cases that have been reliably reported among Malayan fishermen (Reid, 1961; Meldrum and Thompson, 1962).

Quail Myopathy

A very strange myopathy, often fatal, occurs on the island of Lesbos in Greece when the inhabitants eat the flesh of quail, which settle in large flocks on the island during their autumn migration (Billis, Kastanakis, Giamarellou and Daikos, 1971). It is thought that the quail have fed on the seeds of hemlock *Conium maculatum* and that the myopathy is due to poisoning by the alkaloid in hemlock. The condition is not common even on the island of Lesbos, and it is thought that there is an individual susceptibility. Some of the island inhabitants have suffered repeated attacks of the condition while others, equally at risk, have been spared.

Phosphorus Myopathy

A myopathy formerly occurred as an industrial disease in the machine industry of the nineteenth century, but no recent cases have been reported. The condition is reviewed by Adams, Denny-Brown and Pearson (1962), but all the references are to the last century.

References

Adams, R. A., Denny-Brown, D., and Pearson, C. M. (1962). Diseases of Muscle. Hoeber-Harper, New York.

Airaksinen, M. M., and Tammisto, T. (1966). Myoglobinuria after intermittent adminstration of succinylcholine during halothane anesthesia. Clin. Pharmacol. Ther. 7, 583–587.

Begg, T. B., and Simpson, J. A. (1964). Chloroquine neuromyopathy. Brit. Med. J. 1, 770.

Berlin, R. (1948). Haff disease in Sweden. Acta med. scand. 129, 560–572.

Billis, A. G., Kastanakis, S., Giamarellou, H., and Daikos, G. K. (1971). Acute renal failure after a meal of quail. Lancet 2, 702.

Blom, S., and Lundberg, P. O. (1965). Reversible myopathy in chloroquine treatment. Acta med. scand. 177, 685–688.

Blomberg, L. G. (1965). Dystrophia myotonica probably caused by chloroquine. Acta neurol. scand. 41 (Suppl. 13), 647.

Chapman, R. S., and Ewen, S. W. (1969). Chloroquine-induced myopathy. Brit. J. Dermatol. 81, 217–219.

Ebringer, A., and Colville, P. (1967). Chloroquine neuromyopathy associated with keratopathy and retinopathy. Brit. Med. J. 2, 219–220.

Fewings, J. D., Hanna, M. J. D., Walsh, J. A., and Whelan, R. F. (1966). The effects of ethyl alcohol on the blood vessels of the hand and forearm in man. Brit. J. Pharmacol. 27, 93–106.

Garcin, R., Rondot, P., and Fardeau, M. (1964). Sur les accidents neuro-musculaires et en particulier sur une "myopathie vacuolaire" observée au cours d'un traitement prolongé par la chloroquine. Rev. Neurol. (Paris) *111*, 177–195.

Gardner-Medwin, D., and Walton. J. N. (1969). Classification of the neuromuscular disorders. Chapter 13 *in* Disorders of Voluntary Muscle. J. N. Walton (Ed.). Churchill, London.

Golding, D. N., Murray, S. M., Pearce, G. W., and Thompson, M. (1961). Corticosteroid myopathy. Ann. Phys. Med. *6*, 171–177.

Gudden, H. (1896). Klinische und anatomische Beiträge zur Kenntniss der multiplen Alkoholneuritis nebst Bemerkungen über die Regenerations-Vorgänge im peripheren Nervensystem. Arch. Psychiat. Nervenkr. *28*, 643.

Harman, J. B. (1959). Muscular wasting and corticosteroid therapy. Lancet *1*, 887.

Haslock, D. I., Wright, V., and Harriman, D. G. F. (1970). Neuromuscular disorders in rheumatoid arthritis. Quart. J. Med. *39*, 335–358.

Hed, R., Larsson, H., and Wahlgren, F. (1955). Acute myoglobinuria. Report of a case with fatal outcome. Acta med. scand. *152*, 459–463.

Hed, R., Lundmark, C., Wahlgren, F., and Orell, S. (1962). Acute muscular syndrome in chronic alcoholism. Acta. med. scand. *171*, 585–599.

Hicklin, J. A. (1968). Chloroquine neuromyopathy. Ann. Phys. Med. *9*, 189–192.

Hughes, J. T., Esiri, M., Oxbury, J. M., and Whitty, C. W. M. (1971). Chloroquine myopathy. Quart. J. Med. *40*, 85–93.

Jackson, R. C., Bunker, N. U., and Elder, W. J. (1959). Case of carbon-monoxide poisoning with complications. Brit. Med. J. *2*, 1130–1134.

Kahn, L. B., and Meyer, J. S. (1970). Acute myopathy in chronic alcoholism. Amer. J. Clin. Path. *53*, 516–530.

Klinkerfuss, G., Bleisch, V., Diaso, M. M., and Perkoff, G. T. (1967). A spectrum of myopathy associated with alcoholism. II. Light and electron microscopic observations. Ann. Intern. Med. *67*, 493–510.

Lafair, J. S., and Myerson, R. M. (1968). Alcoholic myopathy. Arch. Intern. Med. *122*, 417–422.

Lisander, B. (1970). Myalgia after sulphonamides. Lancet *1*, 1062.

Loftus, L. R. (1963). Peripheral neuropathy following chloroquine therapy. Can. Med. Assoc. J. *89*, 917–920.

Loughridge, L. W., Leader, L. P., and Bowen, D. A. L. (1958). Acute renal failure due to muscle necrosis in carbon-monoxide poisoning. Lancet *2*, 349–351.

Lynch, P. G. (1969). Alcoholic myopathy. J. neurol. Sci. *9*, 449–462.

MacLean, K., and Schurr, P. H. (1959). Reversible amyotrophy complicating treatment with fludrocortisone. Lancet *1*, 701–703.

Martin, J., and Compston, N. (1963). Vincristine sulphate in the treatment of lymphoma and leukaemia. Lancet *2*, 1080–1083.

Mautner, L. S. (1955). Muscle necrosis associated with carbon-monoxide poisoning. A. M. A. Arch. Path. *60*, 136–138.

Meldrum, B. S., and Thompson, R. H. (1962). The action of snake venoms on the membrane permeability of brain, muscle and red blood cells. Guy's Hosp. Rep. *111*, 87–97.

Milligen, K. S., and Suerth, E. (1966). Peripheral neuromyopathy following chloroquine therapy. Med. J. Aust. *1*, 840–841.

Nelson, A. A., and Fitzhugh, O. G. (1948). Chloroquine (SN-7618). Pathologic changes observed in rats which for two years had been fed various proportions. Arch. Path. *45*, 454–462.

Panahi, F., Braun, S., Guiraudon, C., and Delbarre, F. (1968). Deux cas de neuro-myopathie des antimalariques (diagnostic rétrospectif). Bull. Soc. Med. Hosp. Paris *119*, 223–239.

Perkoff, G. T., Diaso, M. M., Bleisch, V., and Klinkerfuss, G. (1967). A spectrum of myopathy associated with alcoholism. I. Clinical and laboratory features. Ann. Intern. Med. *67*, 481–492.

Perkoff, G. T., Silber, R., Tyler, F. H., Cartwright, C. F., and Wintrobe, M. M. (1959). Studies in disorders of muscles. XII. Myopathy due to the administration of therapeutic amounts of 17-hydroxycorticosteroids. Amer. J. Med. *26*, 891–898.

Reid, H. A. (1961). Myoglobinuria and sea-snake-bite poisoning. Brit. Med. J. *1*, 1284–1289.

Renier, J. C. (1965). Apropos du procés-verbal: une observation de neuromyopathie due à l'hydroxychloroquine. Rev. Rhum. *32*, 681–682.

Siemerling, F. (1889). Ein Fall von Alkoholneuritis mit hervorragender Betheiligung des Muskelapparatus nebst Bermerkungen uber das Vorkommen Neuromuscularer Stämmchen in der Muskulatur. Charite-Ann. *11*, 443.

Slotwiner, P., Song, S. K., and Anderson, P. J. (1966). Spheromembranous degeneration of muscle induced by Vincristine. Neurology (Minneap.) *15*, 172–176.

Strandberg, B. (1962). The frequency of myopathy in patients with rheumatoid arthritis treated with triamcinalone. Acta Rheum. Scand. *8*, 31–34.

Valaitis, J., Pilz, C. G., Oliner, H., and Chomet, B. (1960). Myoglobinuria, myoglobinuric nephrosis and alcoholism. Arch. Path. *70*, 195–202.

Weissman, G. (1969). Lysosomes in Biology and Pathology. Vol. I. J. T. Dingle and Honor B. Fell (Eds.). North Holland Publishing Co, Amsterdam.

Whisnant, J. P., Espinosa, R. E., Kierland, R. R., and Lambert, E. H. (1963). Chloroquine neuromyopathy. Proc. Mayo Clin. *38*, 501–513.

Williams, R. S. (1959). Triamcinalone myopathy. Lancet *1*, 698–701.

Yates, D. A. H. (1963). Muscular changes in rheumatoid arthritis. Ann. Rheum. Dis. *22*, 342–347.

Yates, D. A. H. (1970). Steroid myopathy. *In* Muscle Diseases. J. N. Walton, N. Canal and G. Scarlato (Eds.). Excerpta Medica. Amsterdam.

Chapter Eight

Metabolic Myopathies

A large body of research into muscle diseases has been directed to the understanding of the metabolism of muscle and to a search for metabolic abnormalities peculiar to certain muscle diseases. It was hoped that some muscle diseases could be shown to be caused by a single metabolic defect. From such a position of understanding an attempt to correct the metabolic defect might be a feasible method of treatment.

It must be admitted that for the vast majority of muscle diseases no discovery of any specific metabolic explanation of the disease has been made. In particular no causative metabolic defect of the muscle fibre has been found in any of the muscle dystrophies. This failure should not be the cause of dismay, nor should it direct our research into other channels, for what we have learnt about metabolism of muscle strengthens the case for a metabolic explanation of certain muscle diseases. It is significant that the specific enzyme defects that have been related to a muscle disease are examples of enzymes associated with carbohydrate metabolism. We know very much less about the enzymes that are concerned with fat and protein metabolism.

For the reasons given above, what can be reasonably included in a chapter on metabolic diseases of muscle is a matter for discretion. Many myopathies are associated with known metabolic (usually endocrine) diseases, and these puzzling diseases require scrutiny. They will be described under the heading: *myopathies associated with an endocrine disease.* Some rare myopathies have been explained by the absence, or great reduction, of a specific enzyme, either from all organs and tissues or from the muscles alone. These myopathies will be described under the heading: *myopathies due to a known muscle enzyme deficiency.*

Finally there is a group of miscellaneous muscle diseases that are not at present known to have a metabolic basis, but that have significant peculiarities revealed by histochemistry or electron microscopy suggesting a metabolic etiology. These will be described as *miscellaneous myopathies.*

154

MYOPATHIES ASSOCIATED WITH AN ENDOCRINE DISEASE

It is extremely interesting that myopathies have been described as resulting from dysfunction of the pituitary, thyroid, parathyroid and adrenal glands as well as of the endocrine component of the pancreas. The following conditions associated with myopathy will be described here: *Cushing's disease, thyrotoxicosis, hypothyroidism, hyperparathyroidism, periodic paralysis,* and *hyperinsulinsim.*

Cushing's Disease

Overactivity of the pituitary gland causing gigantism or acromegaly does not appear to cause a myopathic state. However, the excessive production of ACTH found in Cushing's disease does appear to cause myopathy.

Cushing's syndrome is caused by an excess of adrenocorticosteroids; the primary defect may be located in the pituitary gland or the adrenals. Many of the features are mimicked by the therapeutic use of steroid drugs in high dosages. The early descriptions of the disease (Cushing, 1932; Plotz, Knowlton and Ragan, 1952) referred to the general tiredness and muscular weakness of which the patients complained. That a distinctive myopathy can occur in the syndrome was reported by Müller and Kugelberg (1959). The myopathy may not respond to treatment by adrenalectomy despite the efficacy of this treatment for the other manifestations of the disease. Prineas, Hall, Barwick and Watson (1968) have suggested that adrenalectomy in Cushing's disease may precipitate the onset of the myopathy.

The clinical picuture of the myopathy is that of excessive tiredness and muscular weakness. There is some tendency to the preferential involvement of proximal muscles but ptosis can also occur. More prominent is the striking fatigue following moderate exertion. The muscles are not tender, and no wasting can be detected.

INVESTIGATIONS

Serum enzymes have been normal, and exercise gives a normal rise of serum lactate levels. There may be the electrolyte disturbance appropriate to Cushing's disease. Myoglobinuria does not appear to have been described. Electromyography demonstrates changes of a myopathy but without specific features. There is spontaneous electrical activity, and increased activity following the insertion of the needle. Pseudomyotonic discharges, fibrillation potentials, and occasional positive sharp waves are found.

PATHOLOGY

Routine examination with conventional histological stains has often shown no abnormality. The most consistent finding has been an increase in the amount of intracellular lipid. Histochemical examination for various muscle enzymes is usually normal. Electron microscopy confirms a conspicuous increase in lipid droplets immediately beneath the sarcolemma and between the myofibrils. Glycogen often appears excessive in the same situations where the fat droplets are found.

Several explantions for the myopathy in Cushing's disease have been advanced. One suggestion is that the electrolyte disturbance (in particular the chronic potassium depletion) is responsible. However, the incidence of myopathy does not appear to correlate with the level of serum potassium, and the myopathy does not respond to potassium therapy. High ACTH production may be the cause; this mechanism of causation would explain why the myopathy may persist or even develop following the successful treatment of the other features of Cushing's syndrome by adrenalectomy. However, a direct effect of the adrenocorticosteroid hormone would also explain many of the features of the myopathy, and the similarity between myopathy in Cushing's disease, human iatrogenic steroid myopathy, and experimental steroid myopathy would thus be explained.

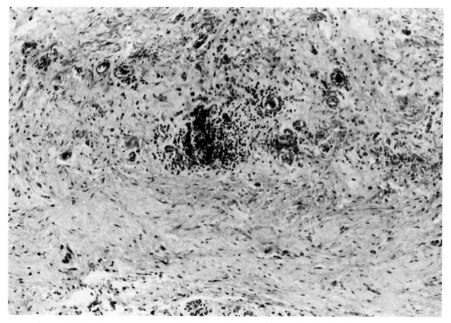

Figure 8–1 Exophthalmic ophthalmoplegia. Biopsy of orbital tissue from a case of severe exophthalmos associated with thyrotoxicosis. Oedema, connective tissue proliferation and lymphocytic infiltration are present. (Haematoxylin and eosin, × 70.)

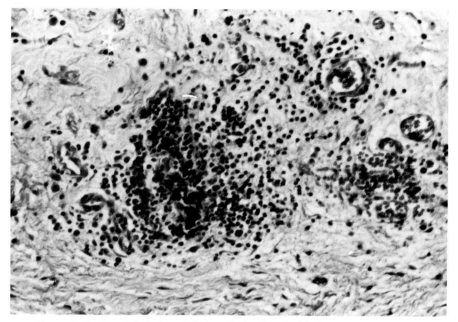

Figure 8–2 Exophthalmic ophthalmoplegia. Detail of inflammatory cell infiltration seen in Figure 8–1. (Haematoxylin and eosin, × 175.)

Thyrotoxicosis

Bathurst (1895) first drew attention to thyrotoxic myopathy in describing a case of exophthalmic goiter complicated by generalised muscular wasting and weakness. Since this early report it has been noted that several types of neuromuscular syndromes can complicate thyrotoxicosis. Starling, Darke, Hunt and Brain (1938) listed these complications as follows: exophthalmic ophthalmoplegia (Figs. 8–1 and 8–2), acute thyrotoxic myopathy, chronic thyrotoxic myopathy, thyrotoxic periodic paralysis, and myasthenia gravis associated with thyrotoxicosis. Of these, only the features of acute and chronic thyrotoxic myopathy will be dealt with in this section. The status even of acute thyrotoxic myopathy is in doubt, as many of the reported cases have been examples of myasthenia gravis. Most reports refer to chronic thyrotoxic myopathy; see Starling *et al.* (1938), Morgan and Williams (1940), McEachern and Ross (1942), Thorn and Eder (1946), Zierler (1951), Quinn and Worcester (1951), Millikan and Haines (1953), Gimlette (1959), Whitfield and Hudson (1961), and Schwartz and Rose (1963).

CLINICAL FEATURES

The condition usually presents with weakness of the muscles of the pelvic girdle; difficulty in climbing stairs and rising from a chair are common early complaints. Even when there is generalised weakness, these muscles are the most severely involved. There may also be weakness of the muscles around the shoulder girdle and of those around the trunk. Less commonly, muscles innervated by the cranial nerves are affected. Subclinical forms of chronic thyrotoxic myopathy are common, judging by the frequency of iliopsoas weakness in thyrotoxicosis and by the findings by electromyography (Havard, Campbell, Ross and Spence, 1963; Ramsay, 1965, 1966).

CLINICAL INVESTIGATIONS

The only important changes are those found by electromyography and those seen in a muscle biopsy. Electromyography has shown a very high incidence of abnormalities (Satoyoshi and Kinoshita, 1970). Shortening of the duration of action potentials, decrease in amplitude, and increase in polyphasic potentials have been found. These abnormalities disappear following successful treatment of the thyroid condition. Increases in the serum creatine and in the amount of creatine in the urine, and a diminished creatine tolerance are all features of thyrotoxicosis and may be related to the effect of the disease on muscle. In the muscle itself, Satoyoshi and Kinoshita found a decrease of creatine phosphate. Water was also diminished, as was potassium, while the sodium was increased.

PATHOLOGY OF THYROTOXIC MYOPATHY

There are conflicting reports on the changes seen in muscle biopsies in thyrotoxicosis, and further studies are required. Some examinations of muscle have shown no abnormality or only minimal changes. A moderate degree of muscle atrophy is the commonest finding. Lymphorrhages have been observed. Rarely there is degeneration of muscle fibres with an increase in the connective tissue and fat.

ETIOLOGY OF THYROTOXIC MYOPATHY

The etiology of thyrotoxic myopathy is at present unknown. The subject is complicated by the cases in which myasthenia gravis or periodic paralysis is associated with thyrotoxicosis. When these cases have been excluded we are left with a group of cases of myopathy with evident clinical weakness and electromyographic changes but without consistent pathological changes. It is likely that the defect in the muscle is not morphological but metabolic, and it has been suggested (Ramsay, 1966) that excessive thyroxine causes "uncoupling" at the stage of oxidative phosphorylation in the mitochondria of muscle.

Hypothyroidism

In addition to the general lethargy and slowness of cretinism and of myxoedema a variety of neuromuscular syndromes may occur in hypothyroidism (Pearce and Aziz, 1969). The disorders of voluntary muscle which may arise in severe hypothyroidism are as follows: pseudo-myotonic syndrome; a syndrome of muscular hypertrophy with pain, weakness and myotonia (the Kocher-Debré-Semelaigne syndrome in cretins and the Hoffman syndrome in adults); a syndrome of muscular cramps suggestive of tetanus; a myasthenic syndrome; and a myopathy which alone will be considered here.

Examples of hypothyroid myopathy have been reported by Alajouanine and Nick (1945), Wilson and Walton (1959), Ästrom, Kugelberg and Müller (1961), Norris and Panner (1966), and by Pearce and Aziz (1969).

CLINICAL FEATURES

The disorder is probably generalised, appears to affect many muscles simultaneously, and is most conspicuous in the larger limb muscles and in the muscles of the trunk. The affected skeletal muscles ache, feel stiff and are subject to cramps. All movement is slow, and frequently slowness of relaxation can be seen. The muscles may show the phenomenon of myoedema in which percussion produces a "dimple" which takes several seconds to fade.

CLINICAL INVESTIGATIONS

Electromyography in hypothyroid myopathy shows a variety of changes, some of which reflect the phenomenon of myotonia that may be present. Electrical "silence" of the muscles in hypothyroidism has been noted (Salick and Pearson, 1967).

PATHOLOGY

The few accounts of the pathological changes in the muscle have given conflicting descriptions. Ästrom *et al.* (1961) described areas of focal necrosis. Asboe-Hansen, Iverson and Wickmann (1952) and Kirchheiner (1962) found subsarcolemmal crescents of homogenous material having the staining properties of acid mucopolysaccharide. Pearce and Aziz (1969) described hypertrophy of individual muscle fibres, some of which showed marked central vacuolation. Necrosis was present in other fibres and regeneration changes were seen. Changes of denervation may be present because a neuropathy frequently coexists with the myopathy.

The ultrastructure of hypothyroid myopathy has been studied in some of the reports quoted above. Foci of myofibrillar damage are present in which the myofibrils are atrophied. The Z bands are affected by widening and "streaming" of Z material into neighbouring parts of the fibre. Sometimes there are rods of Z band material with a structure similar to that seen in "nemaline" myopathy (Godet-Guillain and Fardeau, 1970). Mitochondrial changes are common in which within the cristae are rectangular bodies stratified in parallel sheets. Other inclusions found in the mitochondria are dense and amorphous. Lysosomes and granules of lipofuchsin pigment are prominent. The sarcoplasmic reticulum shows dilatation.

ETIOLOGY OF HYPOTHYROID MYOPATHY

Although the nature of the myopathy is not fully understood, it seems evident that diminution in metabolism due to lack of thyroxine is important. In this context the widespread mitochondrial changes are probably significant. It is of considerable interest that in the experimental animal a state in the muscle is reproduced that is very similar to that seen in the pathology of human cases (Gustafsson, Tata, Lindberg and Ernster, 1965).

Hyperparathyroidism

Weakness, wasting, fatiguability and pain of the skeletal muscles are common in the syndrome of hyperparathyroidism. In the early cases of Hannon, Shorr, McClellan and Dubois (1930) and of Hanes (1939), severe muscle weakness was shown to be a prominent part of the disease.

However, there appears to be a myopathic syndrome which may or may not complicate hyperparathyroidism. Two cases of this syndrome were described by Vicale (1949) among a series of 33 cases of hyperparathyroidism, of which 21 cases complained of muscle weakness. Reports of this myopathic syndrome have appeared by Murphy, Remine, and Burbank (1960), Bischoff and Esslen (1965), Henson (1966), Smith and Stern (1967), and Frame, Heinze, Bolck and Manson, (1968).

CLINICAL PICTURE

The patients suffer from weakness, easy fatiguability, and aching of the muscles, which are hypotonic. The proximal muscles are predominately affected, and there is weakness of the shoulder girdle muscles and a waddling gait. Mental symptoms are often present.

INVESTIGATIONS

The biochemical disturbance of hyperparathyroidism is shown in the blood chemistry. However, there is no direct relationship between the severity of the myopathy and the level of serum calcium. Indeed it is quite possible to have a severe myopathic state in cases of hyperparathyroidism in which the other manifestations are mild. Electromyography has given non-specific features as seen in other myopathies.

PATHOLOGY

There have been few accounts of the histological changes in the affected muscles; the studies that have been made have usually reported minor changes, such as atrophic muscle fibres and fibres undergoing degeneration. The account of Hudson, Cholod and Haust (1970) included observations on the ultrastructure of the muscle, but no specific changes were described.

Periodic Paralysis

Episodes of weakness characterise a disease known as periodic paralysis, which is often familial but may be sporadic. When the disorder was linked to a low plasma potassium, the basis of the disease in causing weakness was thought to be explained. However, the familial form is now known to occur in three types, distinguished by whether the plasma potassium is lowered, elevated or remains normal. The disease is linked to the overproduction of aldosterone by the adrenal gland (Conn, 1955), but this causative mechanism is not operative in all or even most cases.

CLINICAL PICTURE

The patient presents because of attacks of several hours duration in which he experiences flaccid paresis of all four limbs and trunk. Muscles innervated by the cranial nerves are spared, and so the person can talk, swallow and breathe. The condition is inherited as a Mendelian dominant and is most troublesome in the second and third decade, after which it may regress.

CLINICAL INVESTIGATIONS

In the more common hypokalaemic form the plasma potassium is low during an attack, whereas the plasma sodium may be raised. The rapid improvement following the giving of potassium chloride by mouth is helpful in diagnosis.

PATHOLOGY

In early cases and between attacks in severe cases, histological examination of the muscles shows no abnormalities. Commonly, however,

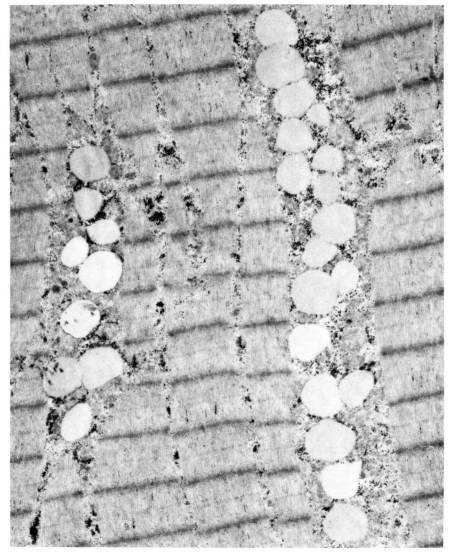

Figure 8–3 Myopathy associated with an inherited disorder of carbohydrate metabolism (Salmon, Esiri and Ruderman, 1971). Electron micrograph of longitudinal section showing central part of a muscle fibre. There are numerous lipid droplets in the intermyofibrillar spaces. (2% aqueous uranyl acetate and lead citrate, × 12,000.)

vacuoles are seen within the muscle fibres; this change is very evident by electron microscopy (Engel, 1966; Howes, Price and Blumberg, 1966). The ultrastructural examination of the muscle fibres shows many lysosomes in relation to the vacuoles, suggesting that muscle fibre degeneration also occurs.

MYOPATHIES DUE TO A KNOWN MUSCLE ENZYME DEFICIENCY

McArdle's Myopathy

In 1951, McArdle (1951) reported the case of a man aged 30 who since childhood had suffered from pain, weakness and stiffness of his muscles following light exercise. While investigating the carbohydrate metabolism of this patient, McArdle noticed that following exercise, there was no rise in the level of blood lactate and blood pyruvate. To explain this he suggested that there was a metabolic defect in that glycogen could not be broken down. The metabolic defect was subsequently shown by Schmid and Mahler (1959) and by Mommaerts, Illingworth, Pearson, Guillory and Seraydarian (1959) to be the absence from the skeletal muscles of the enzyme muscle phosphorylase. McArdle's disease was the first myopathy that was proved to be caused by the absence of a single enzyme. Although the condition is rare, reports of cases have steadily accumulated (Brownell, Hughes, Goldby and Woods, 1969), and many aspects of the disease have now been studied. The condition is inherited as a Mendelian recessive, but sporadic cases are common.

CLINICAL FEATURES

In most cases a routine medical examination would show no abnormality. The history may reveal poor physical performance in childhood and in adolescence, with difficulty in performing moderate exercise because of weakness or cramping pains in the muscles. The specific test of the condition is the performance of muscle exercise under ischaemic conditions. This is most conveniently studied by having the patient exercise the forearm muscles by repeated gripping of the hand while a sphygmomanometer cuff is inflated around the upper arm.

INVESTIGATIONS

The serum levels of creatine phosphokinase and aldolase may be slightly raised. The urine may contain haemoglobin, but in most cases only occasionally, and after severe exertion. The most conclusive investigation is the estimation of serum levels of lactate and pyruvate after exercise, particularly after exercise under ischaemia. In this condition the normal rise of serum lactate and pyruvate after exercise does not occur.

PATHOLOGY

All of our observations on McArdle's disease are based on the biopsy of surgically excised portions of muscle. Relevant information can be obtained on excised muscle by light microscopy, histochemistry, biochemistry and electron microscopy.

LIGHT MICROSCOPY

Paraffin-embedded sections can give satisfactory results but frozen sections retain better the specific abnormalities of the disease. A proportion of the muscle fibres have blebs or vacuoles which are oval, crescentic or circular in shape, and situated at the periphery of the fibre beneath the sarcolemmal sheath (Fig. 8–4). Apart from these blebs or vacuoles, the muscle fibres appear normal. There are no inflammatory or phagocytic cells.

HISTOCHEMISTRY

On frozen sections, PAS staining shows coarse PAS granules. This material can be demonstrated to be glycogen by prior treatment with diastase, which abolishes the positive PAS reaction. Frozen sections incubated for the enzyme phosphorylase demonstrate the absence of the enzyme as compared with control normal muscle, which should be simultaneously treated and examined.

BIOCHEMISTRY

The glycogen content of the freshly excised muscle can be determined as glucose by treating a neutralised perchloric acid extract with diazyme. Values of up to three times that of normal may be obtained. The phosphorylase activity of excised muscle can also be estimated and compared with normal. Details and references to the biochemical methods are given in the paper by Brownell *et al.* (1969).

ELECTRON MICROSCOPY

The muscle fibres show a large excess of glycogen which is conspicuous in the subsarcolemmal regions (Fig. 8–5) but is also prominent between the muscle myofibrils (Fig. 8–6), and may even be seen between individual myofilaments (Fig. 8–7). Apart from the excess of glycogen,

Figures **8–4** to **8–8** illustrate a case of McArdle's myopathy. Examination of portion of excised vastus lateralis muscle from a 17-year-old boy with a congenital deficiency of muscle phosphorylase. (Case of Brownell *et al.*, 1969.)

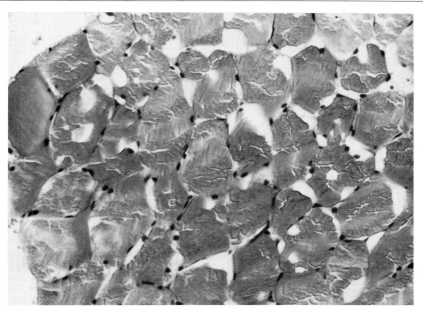

Figure 8–4 McArdle's myopathy. Photomicrograph of transverse section (frozen technique) of muscle, showing the peripheral vacuoles of "blebs." (Haematoxylin and eosin, × 170.)

the muscle fibres show only an increase in lysosomes (Fig. 8–8), indicating that some degeneration of the muscle fibres is taking place. The sarcolemma is elevated over the peripheral blebs of glycogen, which are so prominent by light microscopy.

Phosphofructokinase Deficiency

A clinical syndrome very similar to that seen in McArdle's disease has been described in which the enzyme deficiency has been shown to be that of phosphofructokinase. Cases of this condition have been described by Tarui *et al.* (1965) and by Layzer, Rowland and Ranney (1967).

Other Enzyme Deficiencies

Van Gierke's disease, Pompe's disease and Cori's disease are further examples of disorders of carbohydrate metabolism in which large quan-
(Text continued on page 169.)

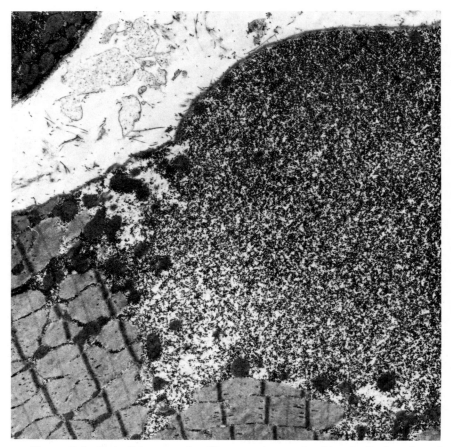

Figure 8–5 McArdle's myopathy. Electron micrograph of longitudinal section of muscle fibre showing the glycogen accumulation in the subsarcolemmal region with elevation of the sarcolemma forming a "bleb." (2% aqueous uranyl acetate and lead citrate, × 14,000.)

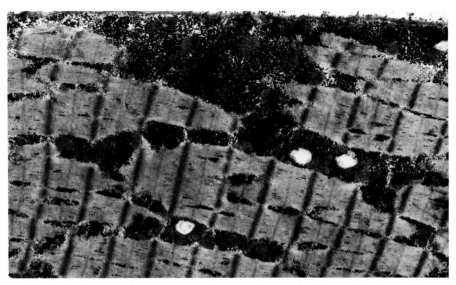

Figure 8–6 McArdle's myopathy. Electron micrograph of longitudinal section showing accumulation of glycogen granules beneath the sarcolemmal sheath and between the myofibrils. (2% aqueous uranyl acetate and lead citrate, × 8000.)

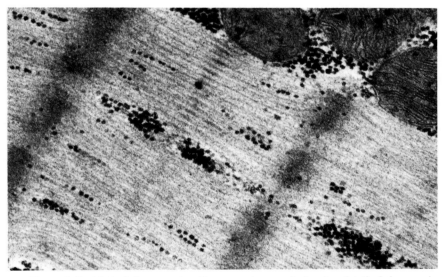

Figure 8–7 McArdle's myopathy. Electron micrograph showing detail of glycogen in sarcomeres seen in longitudinal section. Many glycogen granules are seen between myofilaments. (Lead citrate, × 50,000.)

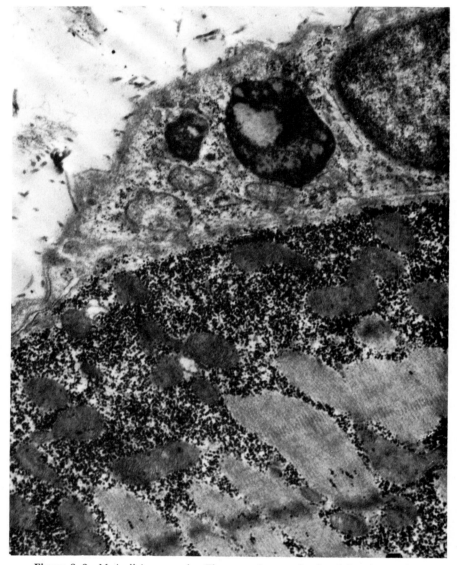

Figure 8–8   McArdle's myopathy. Electron micrograph of peripheral part of a muscle fibre. There is an excess of glycogen with numerous mitochondria. The lysosome is possibly within a satellite cell. (Lead citrate, × 25,000.)

tities of glycogen may be stored in the tissues. In none of these diseases is the enzyme deficiency confined to the skeletal muscles, and so a syndrome of only muscle weakness and cramps does not arise. In Van Gierke's disease, glucose-6-phosphatase is very much reduced in the kidneys and liver, and in these organs there is considerable glycogen accumulation. In Pompe's disease there is a deficiency of α-1, 4-glucosidase, which is normally widely distributed throughout the body. There is widespread glycogen deposition, notably in the heart. In Cori's disease, the enzyme amylo-1, 6-glucosidase is deficient, and there is glycogen storage in the liver, heart and muscles. In all three conditions muscle weakness and hypotonia may by present, but, for the reasons stated, these symptoms are overshadowed by other manifestations.

MISCELLANEOUS MYOPATHIES

Reference will be made to *central core disease, centronuclear myopathy, nemaline myopathy*, and a group of diseases that will be termed *mitochondrial myopathies*.

Central Core Disease

In 1956, Shy and Magee described a new disease in five members from three generations of one family; this condition has become known as *central core disease,* because of the strange morphological appearance of the muscle fibres. The condition is rare and the following list probably includes most of the reported cases: Shy and Magee (1956); Bethlem and Posthumus Meyjes (1960); Seitelberger, Wanko and Gavin (1961); Engel *et al.* (1961); Dubowitz and Platts (1965); Afifi, Smith and Zellweger (1965); Gonatas *et al.* (1965); and Dubowitz and Roy (1970).

GENETICAL STUDIES

Most but not all of the reports have described familial cases spanning two to three generations. All of the family trees published have shown a Mendelial autosomal dominant form of inheritance. No family history was obtained in the single cases reported by Bethlem and Posthumus Meyjes (1960), Engel *et al.* (1961) and Dubowitz and Platts (1965).

CLINICAL FEATURES

The clinical presentation is usually of a mild to moderate non-progressive weakness affecting the lower limbs more than the upper limbs and the proximal muscles more than the distal muscles. The condition may be recognised at any age. Often the normal motor milestones of infancy are correctly achieved, but usually there is some backwardness in activities and sometimes there is aching and stiffness on exercise. Tendon reflexes are usually normal. There are no sensory changes, and intellectual development is normal.

INVESTIGATIONS

The only consistent abnormalities found have been in the electromyogram. The electromyographic findings have been those of a primary myopathy.

PATHOLOGY

All findings so far have referred to the appearance in muscle excised for biopsy. Conventional staining techniques have shown either normal findings or minor changes. Scattered atrophic muscle fibres have been found. The histochemistry of the muscle fibres has proved extremely interesting; this technique is probably essential to making the diagnosis. Using the techniques to demonstrate the enzymes phosphorylase, ATPase and NADH$_2$-TR (Dubowitz and Roy, 1970), the muscle in many of the cases appears to be made up wholly of fibres of type I. The centre of the fibre is negative or weakly stained in these enzyme techniques, so that a "core" is seen. Occasionally in the P.T.A.H. and Masson trichrome stains the "cores" are faintly seen. Sometimes the cores are eccentric but usually they are central, involving about half of the diameter of the muscle fibre. The cores appear to be present only in type I (granular) muscle fibres; the numbers of cores present will depend on the proportion (usually high) of type I fibres, since every type I fibre appears to be affected.

The ultrastructure of the muscle fibre has also proved interesting. The core can readily be distinguished from the peripheral (normal) part of the muscle fibre. Within the core there is disruption of the myofibrillar architecture to an extent which has varied in the reports. Sometimes there is a total disruption but more often there is only a partial alteration. The myofibrils are closely packed, with little interfibrillar space and without mitochondria. The Z line is enlarged, forming many wavy bands of this material.

ETIOLOGY OF CENTRAL CORE DISEASE

As yet the etiology is completely unknown, and there is no evidence at present to regard the disease as a metabolic disease of muscle. The structural changes in the disease have caused much speculation. In foetal development, muscle is of one type until about 20 weeks gestation, at which time granular fibres (type I) appear; by 28 to 30 weeks gestation type I fibres form 50 per cent of the fibres, as in the adult. It has been suggested that the prominence of type I fibres in these cases indicates a fault in muscle development. However, morphological changes similar to the central cores in this disease have been reported from patients with longstanding neurogenic atrophy.

At the moment it is not possible to unite all the data on central core disease into an understanding of the underlying defect in the muscle fibres.

Centronuclear Myopathy (Myotubular Myopathy)

Spiro, Shy and Gonatas (1966) published the case report of a boy aged 12 who throughout his life had shown muscle weakness, particularly of the extraocular and facial muscles. Because of the resemblance of the muscle fibres of their case to the myotubular stage of muscle fibre development in the foetus, the authors named the condition *myotubular myopathy*, and postulated an arrest in the development of the muscle fibre. The preferred name *centronuclear myopathy* refers to the conspicuous finding of numerous central nuclei in the rather small muscle fibres. Many similar sporadic cases of this disease have been described, of which the more recent reports are those of Vital *et al.* (1970) and of Harriman and Haleem (1972). Cases have also been described in which there was a family history of a similar muscle disease. Notable reports of this type are those of Van Wijngaarden, Fleury, Bethlem and Meijer (1969), Bradley, Price and Watanabe (1970) and of Karpati, Carpenter and Nelson (1970).

CLINICAL FEATURES

The families reported have shown a variety of types of inheritance, including dominant, autosomal recessive, and sex-linked inheritance. Except in the family showing sex-linked inheritance (Van Wijngaarden *et al.*, 1969), where 6 males were described, there is no particular sex incidence.

Cases have been described at ages ranging from 1 to 67 years. Usually the condition has been present since infancy. All of the cases have a myopathic state which either is very slowly progressive or is static at a moderate level of disability. The myopathy is seen as weakness of the large muscles of the trunk and limbs, which in most but not all cases is associated with facial muscle weakness and ptosis.

PATHOLOGY

In the first description and in many subsequent reports the muscle fibres have been small, often measuring no more than 20 μ. In other reports there have been two populations of muscle fibres, one of small and one of large muscle fibres. The small fibres have usually been considered to be of histochemical group I and the large fibres of histochemical group II. The muscle fibres have a large central zone of rather empty sarcoplasm, with many large central nuclei and a rim of peripheral myofibrils. This appearance has a resemblance to the myotubule seen in the developing muscle of the foetus.

Electron microscopy shows various degenerating processes occurring in the centre of the muscle fibre. Large amounts of lipofuchsin are found here with lysosomes and autophagic vacuoles. The myofibrils in the centre are often thin or badly formed, and some appear to be degenerating.

The motor innervations of the muscle in this condition appear to be normal as seen by silver techniques or methylene blue impregnation.

ETIOLOGY OF CENTRONUCLEAR MYOPATHY

The pathological appearance of the muscle fibre has been interpreted as a failure of maturation. This would explain the central position of the nuclei and the few myofibrils in the centre of the muscle fibre. It would be reasonable to call this an imperfect maturation rather than an arrest of development. Degeneration of part or all of muscle fibres occurs, but this could be explained as an abnormal susceptibility to degeneration of the imperfect muscle fibres.

Nemaline Myopathy

Shy, Engel, Somers and Wanko (1963) described a congenital non-progressive muscle weakness affecting the proximal muscle groups and characterised by the finding of thread-like rod structures from which they named the disease *nemaline myopathy*.

There have been several subsequent reported cases, of which the following list is a selection: Cohen, Murphy and Donohue (1963); Engel, Wanko and Fenichel (1964); Price *et al.* (1965); Spiro and Kennedy (1965); Hopkins, Lindsey and Ford (1966); Shafiq, Dubowitz, Peterson and Milhorat (1967); Nienhuis *et al.* (1967); and Engel and Gomez (1967).

CLINICAL FEATURES

The cases with a familial incidence suggest an autosomal dominant form of inheritance. Both sexes are affected. There is weakness affecting particularly the proximal limb and trunk muscles. Usually the condition is static, but sometimes there is a slow progression of the weakness. Skeletal deformities including kyphoscoliosis, high arched palate, and an elongated face are common.

PATHOLOGY

There is an increase of fat and connective tissue in the muscle, which may account for 25 per cent of the muscle mass. Actual degeneration of muscle fibres is usually rare. About one-half of the muscle fibres may contain the characteristic rods, but the numbers seen in a single fibre can range from a few to several hundred when a fibre is well seen in longitudinal section. The rods measure up to 5 μ in length and are about 1.5 μ in diameter. They lie within the muscle fibre, concentrated in aggregates often at the poles of the sarcolemmal nuclei. By light microscopy the rods are brilliantly refractile, particularly with phase contrast illumination. They stain with haematoxylin, P.T.A.H., picro-Mallory, and Gomori's trichrome. The study of Nienhuis *et al.* (1967) indicated that the staining properties of the rods were similar to those of tropomyosin B, which is present in the Z bands.

With the electron microscope the rods are seen to be electron dense, with a structure very similar to Z band material. In many fibres the Z bands are abnormal in being locally thickened. Gradations of Z band disorganisation merging to developed rods suggest that the rods originate from Z band material.

ETIOLOGY OF NEMALINE MYOPATHY

Studies of cases of this disease indicate that there is a congenital, probably inherited, disorder of the muscle fibre. Possibly the rods are not specific to this disease, for similar structures have been observed (Fig. 8–9) in muscular dystrophy and in polymyositis (Mair and Tomé, 1972). Also there may be an overlap of some of these inherited myopathies. Afifi, Smith and Zellweger (1965) reported the occurrence of central core disease and nemaline myopathy in members of the same family.

Mitochondrial Myopathies

A number of case reports promise further developments in our understanding of metabolic muscle diseases, and in particular suggest a morphological basis for a biochemical abnormality. In these cases the muscle fibre has been shown to be abnormal, but only because of a structural change of the muscle mitochondria.

Shy, Gonatas and Perez (1966) described under the heading "megaconial myopathy" their finding of large mitochondria containing many rectangular inclusions. They also described a case of "pleoconial myopathy," in which the mitochondria were large, with very numerous cristae often arranged in concentric circles and sometimes containing osmium-dense inclusions. Van Wijngaarden *et al.* (1967) found a defect of oxidative phosphorylation in muscle from a boy of 15 years; the muscle

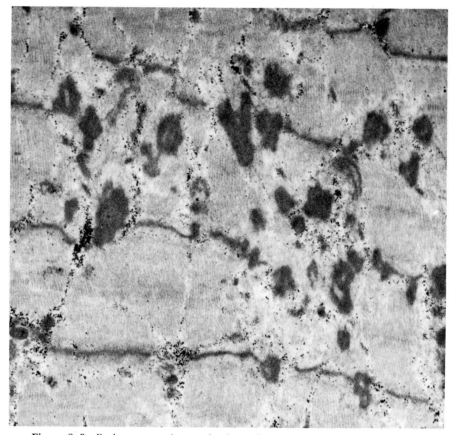

Figure 8-9 Rod structures in muscle. Case of myopathy associated with obstructive jaundice. The electron micrograph shows the peripheral part of a muscle fibre. There are numerous electron-dense structures made up of material similar to that forming the Z line. (2% aqueous uranyl acetate and lead citrate, × 15,000.)

contained very numerous large bizarre mitochondria. The account of Hudgson and Pearce (1969) reviews some of the reports of these interesting mitochondrial abnormalities.

References

Afifi, A. K., Smith, J. W., and Zellweger, H. (1965). Congenital nonprogressive myopathy: central core disease and nemaline myopathy in one family. Neurology (Minneap.) *15*, 371–381.

Alajouanine, Th., and Nick, J. (1945). De l'éxistence d'une myopathie d'origine hypo-thyroidienne. Paris méd. *129*, 346.

Asboe-Hansen, G., Iverson, K., and Wickmann, R. (1952). Malignant exophthalmos; muscular changes and thyrotrophin content in serum. Acta endocrinol. *11*, 376–399.

Åstrom, K. E., Kugelberg, E., and Müller, R. (1961). Hypothyroid myopathy. Arch. Neurol. *5*, 472–482.

Bathurst, L. W. (1895). A case of Graves' disease associated with idiopathic muscular atrophy. Remarks. Lancet *2*, 529–530.

Bethlem, J., Van Gool, J., Hülsmann, W. C., and Meijer, A.E.F.H. (1966). Familial non-progressive myopathy with muscle cramps after exercise. A new disease associated with cores in the muscle fibres. Brain *89*, 569–588.

Bethlem, J., and Posthumus Meyjes, F. E. (1960). Congenital non-progressive central core disease of Shy and Magee. Psychiatr. Neurol. Neurochir. *63*, 246–251.

Bischoff, A., and Esslen, E. (1965). Myopathy with primary hyperparathyroidism. Neurology (Minneap.) *15*, 64–68.

Bradley, W. G., Price, D. L., and Watanabe, C. K. (1970). Familial centronuclear myopathy. J. Neurol. Neurosurg. Psychiat. *33*, 687–693.

Brownell, B., Hughes, J. T., Goldby, F. S., and Woods, H. F. (1969). McArdle's myopathy. A report of a case with observations on the muscle ultrastructure. J. neurol. Sci. *9*, 515–526.

Cohen, P. E., Murphy, E. G., and Donohue, W. L. (1963). Light and electron microscopic studies of "myogranules" in a child with hypotonia and muscle weakness. Can. Med. Assoc. J. *89*, 983–986.

Conn, J. W. (1955). Primary aldosteronism, a new clinical syndrome. J. Lab. Clin. Med. *45*, 6–17.

Cushing, H. (1932). The basophil adenomas of the pituitary body and their clinical manifestations. (Pituitary basophilism). Johns Hopkins Hosp. Bull. *50*, 137–195.

Dubowitz, V., and Platts, M. (1965). Central core disease of muscle with focal wasting. J. Neurol. Neurosurg. Psychiat. *28*, 432–437.

Dubowitz, V., and Roy, S. (1970). Central core disease of muscle: clinical, histochemical and electron microscopic studies of an affected mother and child. Brain *93*, 133–146.

Engel, A. G. (1966). Electron microscopic observations in primary hypokalaemic and thyrotoxic periodic paralyses. Mayo Clin. Proc. *41*, 797–808.

Engel, A. G., and Gomez, M. R. (1967). Nemaline (Z disk) myopathy: observations on the origin, structure, and solubility properties of the nemaline structures. J. Neuropath. Exp. Neurol. *26*, 601–619.

Engel, W. K., Foster, J. B., Hughes, B. P., Huxley, H. E., and Mahler, R. (1961). Central core disease—an investigation of a rare muscle cell abnormality. Brain *84*, 167–183.

Engel, W. K., Wanko, T., and Fenichel, G. M. (1964). Nemaline myopathy: a second case. Arch. Neurol. *11*, 22–39.

Frame, B., Heinze, E. G., Block, M. A., and Manson, G. A. (1968). Myopathy in primary hyperparathyroidism. Ann. Intern. Med. *68*, 1022–1027.

Gimlette, T. M. D. (1959). The muscular lesions in hyperthyroidism. Brit. Med. J. *2*, 1143–1146.

Godet-Guillain, J., and Fardeau, M. (1970). Hypothyroid myopathy. Histological and ultrastructural study of an atrophic form. *In* Muscle Diseases. J. N. Walton, N. Canal, and G. Scarlato (Eds.). Excerpta Medica, Amsterdam.

Gonatas, N. K., Perez, M. S., Shy, G. M., and Evangelista, I. (1965). Central "core" disease of skeletal muscle. Ultrastructural and cytochemical observations in two cases. Amer. J. Path. *47*, 503–515.

Gustafsson, R., Tata, J. R., Lindberg, O., and Ernster, L. (1965). The relationship between the structure and activity of rat skeletal muscle mitochondria after thyroidectomy and thyroid hormone treatment. J. Cell. Biol. *26*, 555–578.

Hanes, F. M. (1939). Hyperparathyroidism due to parathyroid adenoma, with death from parathormone intoxication. Amer. J. Med. Sci. *197*, 85–90.

Hannon, R. R., Shorr, E., McClellan, W. S., and Dubois, E. F. (1930). Case of osteitis fibrosa cystica (osteomalacia) with evidence of hyperactivity of parathyroid bodies; metabolic study. J. Clin. Invest. *8*, 215–227.

Harriman, D. G. F., and Haleem, M. A. (1972). Centronuclear myopathy in old age. J. Pathol. (London) *108*, 237–248.

Havard, C. W., Campbell, E. D., Ross, H. B., and Spence, A. W. (1963). Electromyographic and histological findings in the muscles of patients with thyrotoxicosis. Quart. J. Med. *32*, 145–163.

Henson, R. A. (1966). The neurological aspects of hypercalcaemia: with special reference to primary hyperparathyroidism. J. R. Coll. Physicians (London) *1*, 41–50.

Hopkins, I. J., Lindsey, J. R., and Ford, F. R. (1966). Nemaline myopathy: a long term clinico-pathological study of affected mother and daughter. Brain *89*, 299–310.

Howes, E. L., Price, H. M., and Blumberg, J. M. (1966). Hypokalaemic periodic paralysis: electron microscopic changes in the sarcoplasm. Neurology (Minneap.) *16*, 242–256.

Hudgson, P., and Pearce, G. W. (1969). Ultramicroscopic studies of diseased muscle. *In* Disorders of Voluntary Muscle. 2nd ed. J. N. Walton (Ed.). Churchill, London.

Hudson, A. J., Cholod, E. J., and Haust, M. D. (1970). Familial hyperparathyroid myopathy. *In* Proc. Internat. Cong. Muscle Dis., Milan, 1969. J. N. Walton, N. Canal and G. Scarlato (Eds.). Int. Cong. Ser. No. 199, pp. 526–530. Excerpta Medica, Amsterdam.

Karpati, G., Carpenter, S., and Nelson, R. F. (1970). Type I muscle fibre atrophy and central nuclei. A rare familial neuromuscular disease. J. neurol. Sci. *10*, 489–500.

Kirchheiner, B. (1962). Specific muscle lesions in pituitary-thyroid disorders. Acta med. scand. *172*, 539–543.

Layzer, R. B., Rowland, L. P., and Ranney, H. M. (1967). Muscle phosphofructokinase deficiency. Arch. Neurol. *17*, 512–523.

Mair, W. G. P., and Tomé, F. M. S. (1972). Atlas of the ultrastructure of diseased human muscle. Churchill Livingstone, Edinburgh & London.

McArdle, B. (1951). Myopathy due to defect in muscle glycogen breakdown. Clin. Sci. *10*, 13–35.

McEachern, D., and Ross, W. D. (1942). Chronic thyrotoxic myopathy; a report of 3 cases with a review of previously reported cases. Brain *65*, 181–192.

Millikan, C. H., and Haines, S. F. (1953). The thyroid gland in relation to neuromuscular disease. Arch. Intern. Med. *92*, 5–39.

Mommaerts, W. F. H. M., Illingworth, B., Pearson, C. M., Guillory, R. J., and Seraydarian, K. (1959). A functional disorder of muscle associated with the absence of phosphorylase. Proc. Natl. Acad. Sci. U.S.A. *45*, 791–797.

Morgan, H. J., and Williams, R. H. (1940). Muscular atrophy and weakness in thyrotoxicosis (Thyrotoxic myopathy; exophthalmic ophthalmoplegia). South. Med. J. *33*, 261–268.

Müller, R., and Kugelberg, E. (1959). Myopathy in Cushing's syndrome. J. Neurol. Neurosurg. Psychiat. *22*, 314–319.

Murphy, T. R., Remine, W. H., and Burbank, M. K. (1960). Hyperparathyroidism: Report of a case in which parathyroid adenoma presented primarily with profound muscular weakness. Mayo Clin. Proc. *35*, 629–634.

Nienhuis, A. W., Coleman, R. F., Brown, W. J., Munsat, T. L., and Pearson, C. M. (1967). Nemaline myopathy. A histopathologic and histochemical study. Amer. J. Clin. Path. *48*, 1–13.

Norris, R. H., and Panner, B. J. (1966). Hypothyroid myopathy; clinical, electromyographical and ultrastructural observations. Arch. Neurol. *14*, 574–589.

Pearce, J., and Aziz, H. (1969). The neuromyopathy of hypothyroidism. J. neurol. Sci. *9*, 243–253.

Plotz, C. M., Knowlton, A. I., and Ragan, C. (1952). The natural history of Cushing's syndrome. Amer. J. Med. *13*, 597–614.

Price, H. M., Gordon, G. B., Pearson, C. M., Munsat, T. L., and Blumberg, J. M. (1965). New evidence for excessive accumulation of Z-band material in nemaline myopathy. Proc. Natl. Acad. Sci. U.S.A. *54*, 1398–1406.

Prineas, J., Hall, R., Barwick, D. D., and Watson, A. J. (1968). Myopathy associated with pigmentation following adrenalectomy for Cushing's syndrome. Quart. J. Med. *37*, 63–77.

Quinn, E. L., and Worcester, R. L. (1951). Chronic thyrotoxic myopathy. Report of a case. J. Clin. Endocrinol. Metab. *11*, 1564–1571.

Ramsay, I. D. (1965). Electromyography in thyrotoxicosis. Quart. J. Med. *34*, 255–267.

Ramsay, I. D. (1966). Muscle dysfunction in hyperthyroidism. Lancet *2*, 931–934.

Salick, A. I. and Pearson, C. M. (1967). Electrical silence of myxoedema. Neurology (Minneap.) *17*, 899–901.

Salmon, M. A., Esiri, M. M., and Ruderman, N. B., (1971). Myopathic disorder associated with mitochondrial abnormalities, hyperglycaemia and hyperketonaemia. Lancet *2*, 290–293.

Satoyoshi, E., and Kinoshita, M. (1970). Some aspects of thyrotoxic and steroid myopathy. *In* Muscle Diseases. J. N. Walton, N. Canal and G. Scarlato (Eds.). Excerpta Medica, Amsterdam.

Schwartz, G. A., and Rose, E. (1963). Neuromyopathies and thyroid dysfunction. Arch. Intern. Med. *112*, 555–568.

Schmid, R., and Mahler, R. (1959). Syndrome of muscular dystrophy with myoglobinuria: demonstration of a glycogenolytic defect in the muscle. J. Clin. Invest. *38*, 1040.

Seitelberger, F., Wanko, T., and Gavin, M. A. (1961). The muscle fiber in central core disease. Histochemical and electron microscopic observations. Acta neuropathol. (Berlin) *1*, 223–237.

Shafiq, S. A., Dubowitz, V., Peterson, H. de C., and Milhorat, A. T. (1967). Nemaline myopathy: report of a fatal case, with histochemical and electron microscopic studies. Brain *90*, 817–828.

Shy, G. M., Engel, W. K., Somers, J. E., and Wanko, T. (1963). Nemaline myopathy: a new congenital myopathy. Brain *86*, 793–810.

Shy, G. M., Gonatas, N. K., and Perez, M. (1966). Two childhood myopathies with abnormal mitochondria. I. Megaconial myopathy. II. Pleoconial myopathy. Brain *89*, 133–158.

Shy, G. M., and Magee, K. R. (1956). A new congenital non-progressive myopathy. Brain *79*, 610–620.

Smith, R., and Stern, G. (1967). Myopathy, osteomalacia and hyperparathyroidism. Brain *90*, 593–602.

Spiro, A. J., and Kennedy, C. (1965). Hereditary occurrence of nemaline myopathy. Arch. Neurol. *13*, 155–159.

Spiro, A. J., Shy, G. M., and Gonatas, N. K. (1966). Myotubular myopathy. Persistence of foetal muscle in an adolescent boy. Arch. Neurol. *14*, 1–14.

Starling, H. J., Darke, C. S., Hunt, B. W., and Brain, W. R. (1938). Two cases of Graves' disease with muscular atrophy. Guy's Hosp. Rep. *88*, 117–128.

Tarui, S., Okuno, G., Okura, Y., Tanaka, T., Suda, M., and Nishikawa (1965). Phosphofructokinase deficiency in skeletal muscle. A new type of glycogenosis: an investigation of two dissimilar cases. Biochem. Biophys. Res. Commun. *19*, 517–523.

Thorn, G. W., and Eder, H. A. (1946). Studies on chronic thyrotoxic myopathy. Amer. J. Med. *1*, 583–601.

Van Wijngaarden, G. K., Bethlem, J., Meijer, A. E. F. H., Hülsmann, W. Ch., and Feltkamp, C. A. (1967). Skeletal muscle disease with abnormal mitochondria. Brain *90*, 577–592.

Van Wijngaarden, G. K., Fleury, P., Bethlem, J., and Meijer, A. E. F. H. (1969). Familial "myotubular myopathy." Neurology (Minneap.) *19*, 901–908.

Vicale, C. T. (1949). The diagnostic features of a muscular syndrome resulting from hyperparathyroidism, osteomalacia owing to renal tubular acidosis, and perhaps to related disorders of calcium metabolism. Trans. Amer. Neurol. Assoc., 74th Ann. Meeting, p. 143.

Vital, C., Vallat, J. M., Martin, F., LeBlanc, M., and Bergouignon, M. (1970). Étude clinique et ultrastructurale d'un cas de myopathie centronucléaire (myotubular myopathy) de l'adulte. Rev. neurol. (Paris) *123*, 177–130.

Whitfield, A. G. W., and Hudson, W. A. (1961). Chronic thyrotoxic myopathy. Quart. J. Med. *30*, 257–267.

Wilson, J., and Walton, J. N. (1959). Some muscle manifestations of hypothyroidism. J. Neurol. Neurosurg. Psychiat. *22*, 320–324.

Zierler, K. L. (1951). Muscular wasting of obscure origin and the thyroid gland. Johns Hopkins Hosp. Bull. *89*, 263–280.

Chapter Nine

Miscellaneous Muscle Conditions

Various types of trauma to muscle, the effects of heat, cold and x-rays, vascular disorders of muscle, and tumours peculiar to skeletal muscle will be dealt with in this chapter.

TRAUMA

Trauma to skeletal muscle is a common event in a variety of injuries, but presents no diagnostic difficulty (Figs. 9–1 and 9–2). The extent of repair of the damaged muscle is, however, of considerable importance in the prognosis of cases of injury. Small localised lacerations of muscle heal well, but larger areas of injury, particularly when crushing of muscle has occurred, heal badly, with considerable scar formation. The complications of haemorrhage, loss of blood supply, and sepsis profoundly affect the degree of recovery.

The general response of muscle to injury has been dealt with in Chapter 2; however, some specific forms of muscle trauma merit separate description. These are: *spontaneous rupture of a healthy muscle, rupture of a diseased muscle, muscle haematomas,* and *needle "myopathy."*

Spontaneous Rupture of a Healthy Muscle

This is a surprisingly common condition which occurs in certain occupations and during certain athletic activities. In reviews (Gilcreest, 1925; McMaster, 1933), the occupations mentioned are those of stevedores, baseball players and weight lifters. Many other athletic sports cause the condition, which has also occurred during electro-convulsive therapy and in the convulsions of tetanus.

178

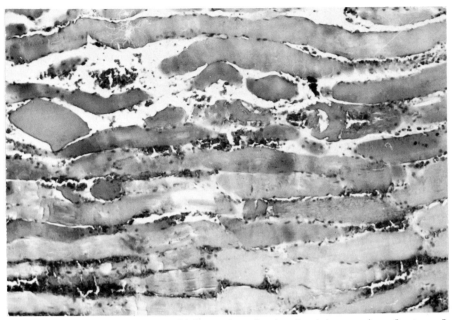

Figure 9–1 Acute trauma. Thigh muscle at the site of an injury causing a fracture of the femur. The muscle fibres seen in the centre of the photomicrograph are torn. There is oedema and haemorrhage in the perimysium. (Haematoxylin and eosin, × 105.)

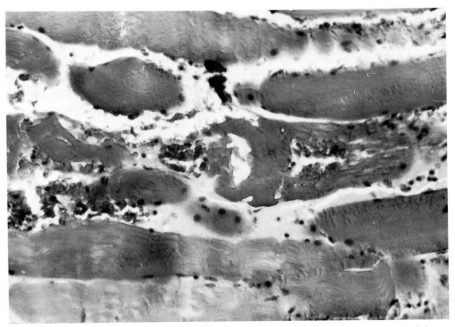

Figure 9–2 Acute trauma. Photomicrograph at higher magnification of same slide as in Figure 9–1 to show detail of the degeneration in the muscle fibres. (Haematoxylin and eosin, × 200.)

The common presentation is the abrupt rupture of the muscle during severe exertion, usually when maximum effort is suddenly applied. Often the rupture is audible, and pain and swelling become quickly evident. The leg muscles are frequently involved, the gastrocnemius being particularly susceptible. A variant of the condition is the rupture of a fascial sheath of a muscle, which causes the muscle to bulge through the fascial tear. The above description refers to the most common presentation but it is not rare for the rupture to occur slowly, causing the complaint of pain, tenderness and swelling, but without the clear history of the condition being caused by violent muscular exercise. Exceptionally the condition presents as a painless soft tissue tumour, but even in these cases the occupation or sport suggests the diagnosis.

The recognition of the distinctive appearance of traumatised muscle is important in those cases without a history of trauma because otherwise a primary muscle disease might be diagnosed. Usually the biopsy obtains not the central area of trauma but a portion of herniated or detached muscle that is undergoing widespread regenerating changes. The muscle fibres are small, stain basophilic, and have many central sarcolemmal neclei. Phagocytes will be present within the muscle if the area is near the trauma. Splitting of the muscle fibre into daughter fibres is often seen, and it is thought that the muscle fibres branch. Ringed fibres can be numerous in traumatised muscle.

Rupture of a Diseased Muscle

The rupture of a muscle at a place weakened by disease differs from the earlier described spontaneous rupture of a healthy muscle. Although a variety of pathological conditions may cause this complication, it has often been described in relation to Zenker's degeneration of muscle. This condition occurs in severe toxaemic states, such as typhoid and typhus fevers, and advanced tuberculosis. The rectus abdominis muscle is most constantly involved, but other abdominal muscles, the abductor thigh muscles, the diaphragm, and the gastrocnemius have all been affected in this way.

Muscle Haematoma

Intramuscular haemorrhage is constantly seen in severe trauma and is particularly evident in bone fractures. The characteristic swelling and tenderness subsides over a period of weeks; in uncomplicated cases the haematoma is completely absorbed without a residual scar. If infection occurs or if the damage to bone and other structures is extensive, fibrosis and contractures will ensue. Intramuscular haemorrhage may also occur from minor trauma in bleeding diseases, particularly haemophilia (Fig.

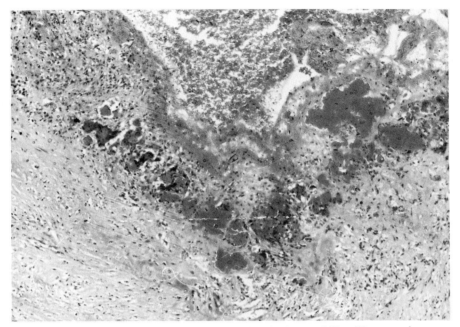

Figure 9-3   Haematoma in the thigh muscle of a haemophiliac. The central upper part of the photomicrograph shows fluid blood. The remainder of the picture shows the thick connective tissue wall of the haematoma cavity. (Haematoxylin and eosin, × 55.)

9-3). The haematoma may continue to enlarge in these conditions and severe disability may result.

Needle "Myopathy"

In the investigation and treatment of many diseases, frequent needling of the larger limb muscles is carried out. It is now well known that recurrent intramuscular needling can cause focal myopathic changes in muscle (Engel, 1967), and this sequel is of importance if part of a muscle at such a traumatised area is excised for a muscle biopsy. This most often happens if electromyographic examination precedes muscle biopsy. The changes seen after a single EMG procedure may be the presence of small foci of muscle fibre destruction seen as muscle fibres undergoing necrosis, phagocytosis of degenerated muscle fibres, and regeneration of damaged muscle fibres. This pattern of muscle damage can present as a histological picture which is interpreted as being due to a natural disease.

With repeated intramuscular injections the pathological changes can be more florid, with a considerable fibrotic reaction (Gray, 1967).

Extensive fibrotic induration with inflammatory changes and sometimes abscess formation can be seen following large numbers of intramuscular injections. This type of muscle damage with sepsis usually arises in drug addicts who administer their drug repeatedly by intramuscular injection (Aberfeld *et al.* 1968).

HEAT, COLD, RADIATION

Various physical agents cause muscle disability. The local destructive effect of heat has been described in Chapter 2. We shall describe here a particular type of myopathy seen in hyperpyrexia. The effects of cold on exposed parts of the body in causing frostbite are well known and do not require detailed description. The information on the effect of x-rays on human muscle is scanty.

Myopathy Associated With Hyperpyrexia

Heat stroke or heat hyperpyrexia is a serious hazard of residence in hot countries and particularly affects untrained persons performing strenuous physical work in a high air temperature. The condition has most often been studied during the training of military personnel in hot countries. What appears to be a similar type of heat stroke occurs during the anaesthetising of certain predisposed individuals. It is now recognised that an important feature in some cases of heat hyperpyrexia is a type of degeneration of skeletal and heart muscle (Vertel and Knochel, 1967), and this has been described in the cases occurring during anaesthesia (Steers, Tallack and Thompson, 1970; Denborough, Ebeling, King and Zapf, 1970). In the cases arising from both these differing circumstances the muscle necrosis becomes evident as myoglobinuria. Impairment of glomerular circulation through the kidney can be caused by the myoglobinaemia, and acute renal failure can result. Susceptibility to this complication of heat hyperpyrexia and anaesthetic hyperpyrexia appears to be inherited as a Mendelian dominant. It may be due to an inherited metabolic defect which is probably a deficiency of intramuscular enzymes.

Frostbite

This is a special form of tissue injury seen in civilians exposed to prolonged very cold temperatures. It is also seen in survivors of shipwreck when these persons have been exposed in life rafts on the sea. In wartime, a variety called "trench foot" or "immersion foot" is seen where campaigns are fought in the trenches of cold countries.

In frostbite the effects on the tissues are brought about by slowing of the circulation. The exposed parts commonly affected are the feet, hands, nose and ears. These parts become white and bloodless but later, if the circulation is re-established, they become red and swollen. The condition is painless during the cold bloodless phase, and this feature is a hazard in that the condition is not quickly recognised.

The pathological findings in frostbite depend on the severity and extent of the tissue damage. In mild cases there is only superficial ulceration of the epidermis, which blisters and desquamates. More severe cases have varying amounts of ischaemic necrosis ranging to gangrene of a whole digit or part of the nose or ear. Following loss of tissue by gangrene, the stump of the digit or the border of the gangrenous area may become permanently hypervascularised. These swollen engorged extremities are frequently painful.

Effect of Radiation on Muscle

Striated muscle is considered to be resistant to the effects of radiation even when relatively high dosages are employed. In clinical practice the effect of diagnostic x-rays on skeletal muscles is considered to be negligible. With therapeutic radiation in high dosages, the effect is thought to be slight, and mainly confined to the neighbourhood of focussed radiation. Rather few clinical observations have been made of the effects of radiation on muscle during cancer therapy, and little fundamental research in experimental animals has been carried out in this field. Nevertheless it would seem that some enquiry into the effects of radiation on muscle is justified, and a review of some of the reports is included here. Hempelmann, Lisco and Hoffman (1952) studied nine cases with the acute radiation syndrome and suggested that the explanation of the weakness and lassitude following therapeutic radiation was a widespread effect on skeletal muscle. This was also the conclusion of Kurohara, Rubin and Hempelmann (1961) from studies on the increased creatinine excretion following radiation therapy.

The early experiments on the effects of radiation on muscle using implanted radium needles were reviewed by Warren (1943). After 40 hours, a zone of necrosis appeared around the needles; these zones were 4 mm in diameter when 5 millicuries was used and 15 mm when 55 millicuries were used. The changes seen in striated muscle following single large doses of x-rays were studied by Lewis (1954). This work was done on rabbits in which the hind limb was given single doses ranging in different animals from 6000 to 72,000 rads. No abnormalities were observed after giving 6000 rads. Destruction of scattered muscle fibres was seen three hours after a single dose of 72,000 rads, and intense necrosis was evident after 12 hours; this progressed over 24 hours to necrosis of most of the leg muscles. Lesser dosages of 36,000; 24,000; and 12,000 showed less severe changes taking longer to manifest themselves.

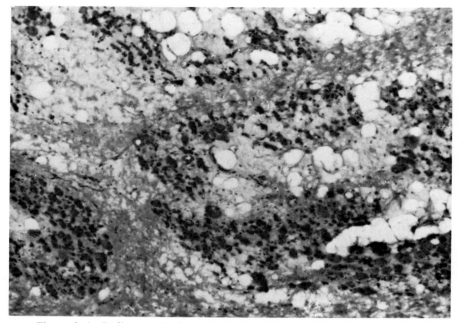

Figure 9–4 Radionecrosis of muscle. Much of the muscle has degenerated and has been replaced by connective tissue and fat. Note the absence of inflammatory reaction. (Haematoxylin and eosin, × 60.)

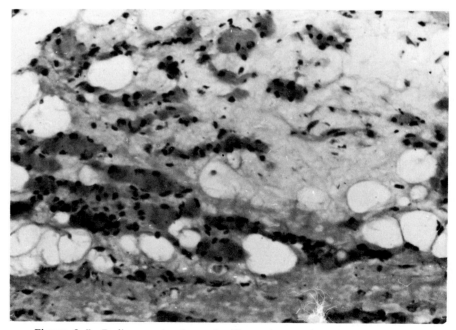

Figure 9–5 Radionecrosis of muscle. Photomicrograph at higher magnification. Vessels are inconspicuous and there are no inflammatory cells. (Haematoxylin and eosin, × 125.)

The changes seen after radiation are those of coagulation necrosis of the muscle fibre cells (Figs. 9–4 and 9–5). The connective tissue and blood vessels are also damaged and haemorrhages occur. Fibroblastic proliferation to repair the damaged muscle is very slow in development. Bergströmm and Salmi (1962) have examined the ultrastructure features of the muscle fibre necrosis and noted the degeneration of the sarcolemma that is produced.

VASCULAR DISORDERS

Some of the vascular disorders affecting muscle have been described elsewhere in this monograph. The important disease *polyarteritis nodosa* is described in Chapter 5. *Gas gangrene*, in which ischaemia contributes to the extension of the condition, is described in Chapter 6. *Frostbite* has been described earlier in this chapter. Remaining to be considered are the syndromes of chronic and acute ischaemia of muscle. The latter is also known as *Volkmann's ischaemic contracture* (Figs. 9–6 to 9–9) when the condition complicates a limb fracture.

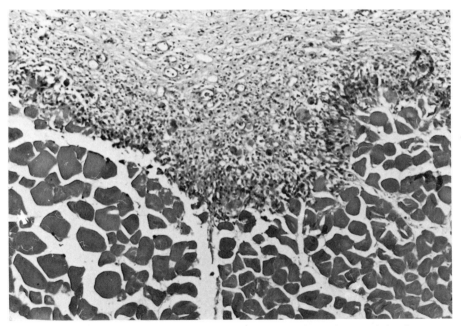

Figure 9–6 Volkmann's ischaemic contracture. The photomicrograph is of a transverse section of muscle form an amputated limb in which a fracture had caused obstruction to the major limb artery. The upper part of the picture shows the margin between granulation tissue (*above*) and surviving muscle (*below*). Note the regeneration by the sprouting of muscle fibres which attempt to grow into the fibrous tissue. (Haematoxylin and eosin, × 65.)

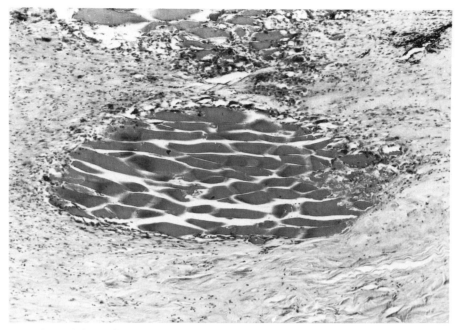

Figure 9–7 Volkmann's ischaemic contracture. Photomicrograph of a longitudinal section through severely affected leg muscle. The picture shows a surviving portion of muscle surrounded by granulation tissue. Note the evidence of regeneration at all parts of the margin of the muscle. (Haematoxylin and eosin, × 50.)

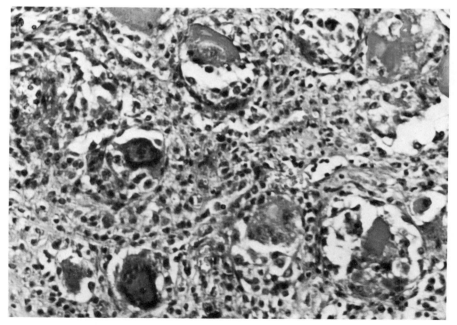

Figure 9–8 Volkmann's ischaemic contracture. Photomicrograph of a transverse section at the regenerating margin of the muscle. Note the regenerating muscle fibres which in transverse section give the appearance of multinucleated giant cells (Haematoxylin and eosin, × 160.)

186

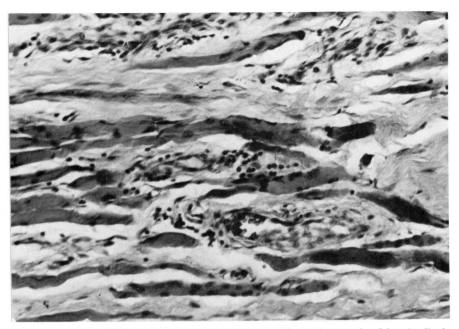

Figure 9–9 Volkmann's ischaemic contracture. Photomicrograph of longitudinal section showing regenerating muscle fibres at growing margin of surviving muscle. (Haematoxylin and eosin, × 145.)

Chronic Ischaemia of Muscle

Atherosclerosis is the commonest disease of major arteries and in elderly persons will commonly be present in all the major limb arteries. In some of these cases the iliac and femoral arteries will have been gradually stenosed over some years, possibly with occasional more sudden occlusion due to thrombosis. It would seem that this arterial pathology would cause a chronic ischaemic effect throughout the skeletal muscles of the limb concerned. Very little attention has been paid to this type of chronic muscle ischaemia. However, it may explain part of the frailty and inactivity forced upon elderly persons.

Acute Ischaemia of Muscle

Sudden ischaemia of muscle usually affects a whole limb and commonly one lower limb or its extremity. The commonest cause is an embolus lodging in the femoral artery or one of its branches. Initially the limb is pale, cold and swollen. There may be paraesthesia or loss of sensation. If the direct circulation is not quickly restored or if a collateral circulation is not established, irreversible changes will occur in the limb.

The tissue becomes discoloured as the result of tissue death, and the limb becomes initially yellow and later black. The pathological findings in the muscle following acute ischaemia have been described in Chapter 2.

TUMOURS

Both primary and secondary tumours are uncommon in human skeletal muscle. The primary tumours can be subdivided into a group of tumours arising from muscle fibre cells and a second group consisting of those tumours arising from other constituents of the muscle belly. There are three examples of tumours arising from muscle cells: The *rhabdomyoma*, the *rhabdomyosarcoma* and the *granular-cell myoblastoma*. However, the cell of origin of the last named tumour is open to question.

Rhabdomyoma

According to Stout and Lattes (1967), not more than 12 cases of this type of tumour have been reported. These 12 tumours were found in the tongue, neck muscles, larynx, uvula, nasal cavity and vulva. The tumours have been encapsulated masses of benign behaviour. Microscopically they have consisted of either rounded or somewhat elongated cells with peripheral nuclei. Striations in the cells are essential for the diagnosis; sometimes there are long, interdigitating, spindle-shaped cells giving the appearance of adult muscle cells. Mitoses have not been seen, and at the margin of the tumour the surviving tissue is not invaded in the manner of a malignant tumour.

The description above refers to the very rare examples arising in human skeletal muscle. The so-called rhabdomyoma arising in the heart is much commoner but appears to be a malformation rather than a true tumour. It has a distinctive appearance of large plump cells filled with glycogen vacuoles.

Rhabdomyosarcoma

These tumours can be separated into adult and juvenile types. The adult form tends to be found in the deeper tissues of the limbs and the trunk, whereas the juvenile form is found in the head and neck and in the urogenital region (Stout and Lattes, 1967). The macroscopical appearance is that of a deep-seated tumour usually situated within muscle but often involving other tissues, or presenting, particularly after incomplete surgical excision, through the skin. Local infiltration is common, and the tumour may metastasise, usually by haematogenous and less commonly by lymphocytic channels.

The microscopical appearance of the rhabdomyosarcoma (Figs. 9–10 and 9–11) is variable, and the characteristic rhabdomyoblasts are not easy to identify with certainty. Stout and Lattes suggest that the rhabdomyoblast may be:

1. a rounded or strap-like cell with two adjacent nuclei,
2. a racket-shaped cell with a single nucleus in the large expanded part,
3. a small rounded uninucleate cell, or
4. a giant multinucleated cell.

The tumour cells often have vacuolar structures containing glycogen. The cytoplasm is eosinophilic and occasionally shows cross striations or longitudinally oriented structures with the appearance of myofibrils.

The juvenile rhabdomyosarcomas can have a macroscopical and microscopical appearance similar to the adult form, but in certain regions such as the pharynx, nasal cavity and urogenital region (sarcoma botryoides), they have distinctive features of great interest in tumour classification but outside the scope of this account of muscle pathology.

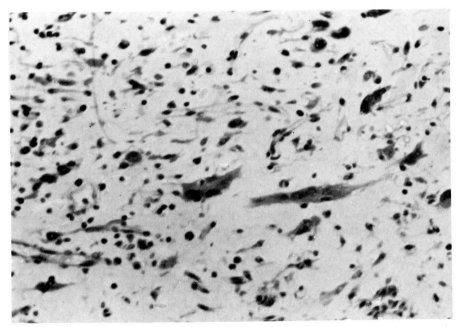

Figure 9–10 Rhabdomyosarcoma. Photomicrograph of a section from a deep-seated malignant tumour of the lower limb. The tumour cells are variable in size and shape but most have a spindle-like form. Multinucleated tumour cells resembling muscle fibres are not common. (Haematoxylin and eosin, × 60.)

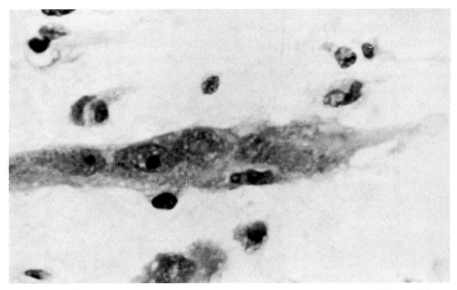

Figure 9–11   Rhabdomyosarcoma. Photomicrograph showing one of the multinucleated cells in Figure 9–10 at higher magnification. (Haematoxylin and eosin, × 220.)

Granular Cell Myoblastoma

A detailed account will not be given of these interesting tumours, because their origin from myoblasts has never been proved. The original accounts of Abrukossoff were of tumours located in voluntary muscle and particularly found in the tongue. Subsequently many examples have been reported from diverse sites, including the skin and mucosae, which do not contain skeletal muscle. The subject of the origin of these tumours has recently been revived by the application of modern techniques. Electron microscopy (Fisher and Wechsler, 1962), tissue culture (Murray, 1951), and histochemistry (Pearse, 1950) have given conflicting evidence, but none in favour of an origin from myoblasts. Macroscopically these tumours are usually small circumscribed tumors of slow growth, but a malignant variety also occurs. The microscopical appearance is that of a tumour made up of large, polygonal, sometimes spindle-shaped cells with abundant cytoplasm, having numerous fine eosinophilic granules (Powell, 1946).

Other Primary Tumours Arising in Skeletal Muscle

Angiomas are relatively common in muscle, where their features do not differ from such malformations elsewhere. *Fibromas* and the similar

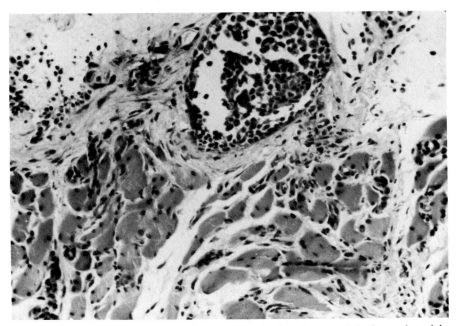

Figure 9–12 Secondary carcinoma. Metastasis of carcinoma of the breast into deltoid muscle excised for biopsy. (Haematoxylin and eosin, × 70.)

desmoid tumours are also found. The malignant tumour found in muscle is the *fibrosarcoma*.

Secondary Tumours in Muscle

Secondary tumours are considered to be rare in skeletal muscle, except for the direct invasion of neighbouring muscle that commonly occurs in relation to a malignant tumour. Metastatic tumours are rarely seen in skeletal muscle, although they may be commoner than is realised (Fig. 9–12). Pearson (1959) found six examples of metastatic tumour out of 38 cases of malignant disease surveyed at necropsy.

References

Aberfeld, D. C., Bienenstock, H., Shapiro, M. S., Namba, I. T., and Grab, D. (1968). Diffuse myopathy related to meperidine addiction in a mother and daughter. Arch. Neurol. *19*, 384–388.

Bergströmm, R. M., and Salmi, A. (1962). Radiation-induced damage in the ultrastructure of striated muscle. Exp. Cell Res. *26*, 226–228.

Denborough, M. A., Ebeling, P., King, J. O., and Zapf, P. (1970). Myopathy and malignant hyperpyrexia. Lancet *1*, 1138–1140.

Engel, W. K. (1967). Focal myopathic changes produced by electromyographic and hypodermic needles ("needle myopathy"). Arch. Neurol. *16*, 509–511.

Fisher, E. R., and Wechsler, H. (1962). Granular cell myoblastoma — a misnomer. Electron microscopic and histochemical evidence concerning its Schwann cell derivation and nature (granular cell schwannoma). Cancer *15*, 936–954.

Gilcreest, E. L. (1925). Rupture of muscles and tendons, particularly subcutaneous rupture of the biceps flexor cubiti. J.A.M.A. *84*, 1819–1822.

Gray, J. E. (1967). Local histologic changes following long-term intramuscular injections. Arch. Path. *84*, 522–527.

Hempelmann, L. H., Lisco, H., and Hoffman, J. G. (1952). The acute radiation syndrome: a study of nine cases and a review of the problem. Ann. Intern. Med. *36*, 279–510.

Kurohara, S. S., Rubin, P., and Hempelmann, L. H. (1961). Creatinuria and fatigue in patients undergoing radiation therapy. Radiology *77*, 804–812.

Lewis, R. B. (1954). Changes in striated muscle following single intense doses of x-rays. Lab. Invest. *3*, 48–53.

McMaster, P. E. (1933). Tendon and muscle ruptures. J. Bone Joint Surg. (Br.) *15*, 705–722.

Murray, M. R. (1951). Cultural characteristics of three granular-cell myoblastomas. Cancer *4*, 857–865.

Pearse, A. G. E. (1950). Histogenesis of granular-cell myoblastoma (? granular-cell perineural fibroblastoma). J. Path. Bact. *62*, 351–362.

Pearson, C. M. (1959). The incidence and type of pathological alterations observed in muscles in routine autopsy survey. Neurology (Minneap.) *9*, 757–766.

Powell, E. B. (1946). Granular cell myoblastoma. Arch. Path. *42*, 517–524.

Steers, A. J. W., Tallack, J. A., and Thompson, D. E. A. (1970). Fulminating hyperpyrexia during anaesthesia in a member of a myopathic family. Brit. Med. J. *1*, 341–343.

Stout, A. P., and Lattes, R. (1967). Tumours of the Soft Tissues. Fascicle 1. Second Series. Atlas of Tumour Pathology. Armed Forces Institute of Pathology, Bethesda, Maryland.

Vertel, R. M., and Knochel, J. P. (1967). Acute renal failure due to heat injury. Amer. J. Med. *43*, 435–451.

Warren, S. (1943). Effects of radiation on normal tissues. XIV. Effects on striated muscle. Arch. Path. *35*, 347–349.

Chapter Ten

Investigation of Muscle Diseases

The elucidation of a case of suspected muscle and neuromuscular disease may require the collaboration of several specialists, each contributing a part to the total investigation of the patient. The purpose of this chapter is to indicate the variety and scope of the investigations available. Not all of the measures discussed here will be applicable to every case of suspected muscle or neuromuscular disease; an individual case, for example, of *dystrophia myotonica* might be correctly diagnosed on clinical grounds alone. But commonly a muscle disease presents as a diagnostic problem for which several investigations are needed. In the United Oxford Hospitals we have developed in the past ten years a regime of investigation combining clinical evaluation with biochemical investigations, electrophysiological recordings, and the interpretation of muscle biopsies.

These separate methods of investigation will now be considered under the following headings: Clinical Aspects, Electrophysiological Methods, Biochemistry, and Muscle Biopsy. Some histological technical methods will be included at the end of the chapter.

CLINICAL ASPECTS

The clinical examination of these cases is divided into the taking of the clinical history of the case (and of the family history where this is appropriate) and the performance of a detailed clinical examination.

Clinical History

The three main types of symptoms of muscle disease are *weakness, pain* and *changes of muscle tone.*

193

The mode of onset and the distribution of the muscle weakness is of considerable importance. Commonly the weakness is slow in onset and gradually progressive, but in periodic paralysis it may be intermittent, alternating with periods of complete recovery. Weakness following exercise but relieved by rest is characteristic of myasthenia gravis. The distribution of the muscle weakness differs widely. The shoulder and limb muscles are predominantly affected in some of the muscle dystrophies, whereas in motor neurone disease the small muscles of the hands and feet are conspicuously involved in the earlier stages.

Pain in muscle disease can be of several types. In neurological diseases causing upper motor neurone paresis, the flexor spasms associated with the spastic paresis can be painful. In poliomyelitis and in polyneuritis the onset of the condition is often painful. When there is hyperexcitability of the neuromuscular apparatus, as in tetany and tetanus, the muscle spasms thus produced can be very painful. Pain is conspicuous in certain muscle diseases of which *Bornholm disease, polymyositis, polyarteritis nodosa* and *polymyalgia rheumatica* deserve mention.

Pain arising during muscular exertion differs from the type already discussed. The commonest form is severe pain in the lower limbs, seen as the intermittent claudication of extensive vascular disease. Rarely, painful cramps occurring only on exercise are due to the congenital myophosphorylase deficiency disease known as McArdle's disease.

Changes of muscle tone may be manifest as a diminution or an increase; such changes are more likely to be found on clinical examination than known to the patient.

Family History

Several muscle and neuromuscular diseases are inherited, and special enquiry should be directed to obtaining a reliable family history. Sometimes investigations can be more conveniently carried out on a parent or sibling suffering from the same inherited disease. Some information on the common inherited muscle and neuromuscular diseases will be given here. For a fuller account the reader is referred to Pratt (1967) and to Kloepfer and Emery (1969).

INHERITED DISEASES

WERDNIG-HOFFMANN DISEASE (infantile progressive spinal muscular atrophy) was extensively investigated by Brandt (1951), who found data from 52 sibships indicating an autosomal recessive form of inheritance.

KUGELBERG-WELLANDER DISEASE (juvenile progressive spinal muscular atrophy) has usually been reported with data suggesting an autosomal recessive inheritance (Kugelberg and Welander, 1956).

FAMILIAL MOTOR NEURONE DISEASE occurs in a dominantly inherited form (Kurland and Mulder, 1955) of which about 40 families have been recorded. On the island of Guam familial motor neurone disease occurs in a form associated with Parkinsonism and dementia, and is usually referred to as the *Parkinsonism-dementia complex.* (Hirano, Kurland, Krooth and Lessell, 1961; Hirano, Malamud and Kurland, 1961).

MUSCULAR DYSTROPHIES: The inheritance of the muscular dystrophies is a complex subject because of the disputed classification of some varieties. Only the principal forms will be listed here. *Duchenne dystrophy* is, with rare exceptions, seen only in boys, in which it is inherited as a sex-linked recessive character. *Facioscapulohumeral muscular dystrophy* is inherited as an autosomal dominant character. *Limb girdle dystrophy* is mainly inherited as a recessive, with some observations suggesting a dominant inheritance. *Dystrophia myotonica* appears to be dominantly inherited.

FAMILIAL PERIODIC PARALYSIS appears to be caused by dominant inheritance, and McARDLE'S DISEASE appears to be inherited as a recessive.

Clinical Examination

The main physical signs of muscle and neuromuscular disease are weakness, atrophy and hypertrophy of muscles, disturbance of muscle tone, and fasciculation. In addition there may be many signs of involvement of the nervous system or other systems relevant to the case.

Weakness as a physical sign amplifies the information gained in taking the clinical history. The distribution of the muscle weakness often provides important information.

Muscle tone is notably diminished in many muscle diseases and is particularly seen in the muscle dystrophies of childhood. The "floppy infant" refers to the diagnostic problem posed by a weak hypotonic child. *Hypertonia* is usually caused by the spasticity of upper motor neurone paresis and is present frequently in neuromuscular disease. More important is *myotonia,* a failure of muscle to relax after contraction; this is present in Thomsen's disease.

Fasciculation is caused by the simultaneous contraction of small groups of muscle fibres, usually those forming a single motor unit. It is seen as movement of the skin by the underlying muscle. This sign indicates a disorder of the motor neurone and is well seen in motor neurone disease. It is not present in primary muscle diseases.

ELECTROPHYSIOLOGICAL METHODS

Only a brief outline of electrophysiological methods will be given here. For further information readers are referred to the accounts of Licht (1961), Norris (1963), Ruch, Patton, Woodbury and Towe (1965), Cohen and Brumlik (1968) and Lenman and Ritchie (1970).

The two most helpful diagnostic techniques are electromyography and nerve conduction studies.

Electromyography

In this technique needle electrodes are inserted into the muscle to be examined. These needle electrodes may be coaxial or monopolar. A *coaxial* needle electrode is made up of a fine hollow needle into which is inserted a solid needle covered by a layer of insulation along its length. The electrical potentials between the inner and outer needles are measured by a recording on an oscilloscope; they are "heard" by audio amplifiers through a loud-speaker.

The *monopolar* electrode consists of a single solid needle coated with insulation up to the naked tip. This single electrode detects potential difference with greater clarity, but emanating from a larger radius than recordings from a coaxial electrode.

Normally the activity of the muscle is evaluated by a skilled observer watching the oscilloscope and listening to the loud speaker. A permanent record can be made by photographing the pattern of the electrical potentials, but usually only a limited portion of tracing can be recorded. The use of a tape recorder enables long recordings to be made and permits computer analysis of recordings.

The electrical activity of the chosen muscle is examined *during insertion of the electrode, with the muscle resting* and *with the muscle performing work*. The amplitude, duration, wave form and frequency of the potentials obtained are studied. On insertion of the electrode into the muscle, a short burst of electrical activity occurs which may last 0.5 second and may be from 50 to 150 μV in amplitude. At rest the muscle should give no electrical activity. On contraction of the muscle, motor unit potentials are obtained; the number and strength of these indicates the activity of the muscle.

In muscle and neuromuscular diseases, the motor unit potentials may be abnormal in being either increased or decreased in amplitude, frequency and duration. Increase in amplitude and duration of motor unit potentials is seen in diseases of the anterior horn cell. Small motor unit potentials of short duration are seen in primary muscle disease. *Fasciculation* (the spontaneous contraction of an individual motor unit) and *fibrillation* (the spontaneous contraction of an individual muscle fibre) can be recognised by the characteristic motor unit potentials.

Nerve Conduction Studies

A variety of techniques of studying nerve conduction are now available, most consisting of the measurement of the times of the conduction of nerve impulses. If the peripheral trunk of a motor nerve is stimulated by a skin electrode, a contraction is obtained in the muscle supplied. The time interval between stimulus and contraction is called the latency time, or conduction time. The speed of the nerve impulse is slower at the termination of the nerve; for this reason, conduction velocity along nerve trunks is measured by observing the effects of electrical stimulation at two separate points along the nerve. By measuring the two conduction times and by subtraction, the time elapse of traversing the nerve between the two different points of stimulation can be calculated. The conduction velocity of the nerve trunk is expressed in metres per second.

Conduction studies on sensory nerves are performed by stimulating the nerves by cathode and anode electrodes placed near them while recordings are made from an electrode placed higher up (orthodromic) or lower down (antidromic) the sensory nerve trunk. Several other techniques using nerve conduction studies are available, but the only one to be mentioned here is the demonstration of fatigability. Neuromuscular fatigability of the neuromuscular unit can be demonstrated by repetitive stimulation. By this means subclinical myasthenia gravis or the myasthenic syndrome can be detected.

BIOCHEMISTRY

Several biochemical estimations on urine, blood or excised muscle have a place in diagnosis of muscle diseases, but the most valuable are the levels of certain serum enzymes.

Urine Estimations

Creatine and creatinine and certain amino acids are present in urine in abnormal amounts in certain muscle diseases. Normally there is no creatine in the urine, but creatinine is excreted in amounts ranging from 1 to 2 g per day. In diseases with increased muscle breakdown, creatine and creatinine excretion is very much higher. The highest figures are obtained in muscle dystrophy, with smaller elevations noted in denervations and polymyositis. (Van Pilsum and Wolin, 1958).

The development of the technique of paper chromatography of urine has enabled the indentification and the approximate measurement of amino acid excretion. Normally small quantities of several amino acids are excreted. In muscle dystrophies and in some other muscle diseases (Pennington, 1969) certain amino acids are present in the urine in increased amounts.

Serum levels of certain muscle enzymes become elevated in diseases in which muscle fibre destruction is common. The most useful enzymes in diagnosis and prognosis are serum creatine phosphokinase and serum aldolase. The following enzymes also may appear in increased amounts: aspartate aminotransferase (GOT),* alanine aminotransferase (GPT),† lactate dehydrogenase, glucose phosphate isomerase, phosphoglycomutase, α hydroxybutyrate dehydrogenase, and malate dehydrogenase (Pennington, 1969).

Serum creatine phosphokinase (CPK) was shown by Ebashi, Toyokura, Momoi and Sugita (1959) to be greatly raised in muscular dystrophy, and we now recognise that this enzyme level is the most accurate measure of many muscle diseases. The enzyme transfers a phosphate group from creatine phosphate to A.D.P., forming creatine and ATP. If the measurement is carried out on this reaction (the reverse reaction also occurs), the result can be expressed as the amount of creatine formed per hour per ml of serum at 37°C. Normal persons have up to 60 international units per litre. In childhood muscle dystrophy, the serum creatine phosphokinase level may be several hundred times the normal. In the less severe adult dystrophies the serum levels are less, but are still very high. In polymyositis the levels are usually those of moderate to marked increase, according to the activity of the disease. Denervation of muscle causes little or no increase.

In addition to the value of this enzyme determination in diagnosis, the levels have considerable importance in assessing the activity of the disease. Also, the symptomless carriers of Duchenne dystrophy (the mothers of the affected boys of this sex-linked disease) show moderate elevation of this serum enzyme.

Aldolase is a widespread tissue enzyme which catalyses the breakdown of fructose 1:6-diphosphate. It was discovered by Sibley and Lehninger (1949) that high levels of this enzyme appear in the blood in active cases of muscle dystrophy. The elevation is most notable in the early stages of Duchenne dystrophy. The levels may be only slightly raised or normal in adult types of dystrophy and in dystrophia myotonia. In polymyositis there is a rise, the amount of which depends on the activity of the disease. Normal levels (up to 10 units) are obtained in denervating conditions and in myasthenia gravis.

MUSCLE BIOPSY PROCEDURES

The histological examination of a portion of surgically excised muscle can be of great assistance in the diagnosis of an individual case, but only if some thought is given to the selection of the patient and of the muscle sampled.

---

*called also *glutamic-oxalacetic transaminase*
†called also *glutamic-pyruvic transaminase*

Safety of Muscle Biopsy

Excision of portions of muscle from major proximal limb muscles seldom causes any added disability. Muscle regenerates rapidly; in experimental work, excised muscle has usually been replaced in about 2 months. Even in human denervating diseases and in primary muscle diseases, regeneration proceeds rapidly. Having stated this favourable sequel to muscle excision, one must also sound a warning against indiscriminate biopsies, particularly of small muscles or of the muscles of children. The careful clinical consideration of each case is important; trouble usually arises by thoughtless adherence to a standard procedure inappropriate to an individual case. The only major hazard in taking a muscle biopsy is sepsis, but this complication should never occur if the operation of excision is regarded as a surgical procedure demanding all the usual precautions of an open operation.

Selection of Patient

Failure to obtain useful information from a muscle biopsy is often due to the procedure being performed in cases unlikely to show changes. The most likely diagnosis to be resolved is the etiology of a progressive muscular wasting. The distinction between primary muscle disease and denervating diseases is often easy by muscle biopsy. In general, widespread denervating disease always gives appropriate changes, muscular dystrophies have usually severe changes, collagen diseases may sometimes reveal the diagnosis, and in the metabolic or toxic myopathies changes may be slight or only revealed by special techniques.

Selection of Muscle

The choice of an appropriate muscle from which a portion may be surgically excised is very important. Electromyography is useful in assessing the severity of involvement of a muscle, but the biopsy should never be taken from the actual site of the electromyography. The muscle selected should be clearly affected by the disease, but not be atrophic, when it may consist only of fat and connective tissue. For technical reasons it is desirable to choose a muscle or that part of a muscle in which the fibres are running parallel, so that transverse and longitudinal sections may be easily oriented. The following muscles are suitable: deltoid, pectoralis major, biceps brachii, brachioradialis, palmaris longus, rectus abdominis, intercostal muscle, rectus femoris, vastus lateralis, tibialis anterior, peroneus longus, and peroneus brevis.

These examples are of large and convenient muscles, but others technically suitable could be mentioned. The small intrinsic muscles of the hands and feet, the muscles innervated by the cranial nerves, and particularly the extraocular muscles yield excellent sections when, as at necropsy, they can be examined. Opportunities should be taken to excise a portion of muscle during some other operative procedure which may provide an adequate portion of muscle and eliminate the need for a second operation. Orthopaedic operations to correct joint deformities are examples. Thymectomy for myasthenia gravis enables neighbouring muscle to be obtained. Some diseases have localised disability; in these cases, choosing the correct muscle to examine requires especially careful consideration. In collagen diseases, affected muscle may be tender, and the site of tenderness may be a guide to the appropriate muscle.

In all biopsies it is of considerable advantage to examine a portion of muscle that includes the terminal innervation; this is essential in diseases such as myasthenia gravis and the acute neuropathies. The motor "point" area is usually situated halfway between the origin and insertion of a muscle, and is a broad zone rather than a point. Nevertheless, care must be taken not to excise too much of the motor point area. It is safe if the recommended procedure is followed of excising a rectangular portion of muscle oriented longitudinally. The localisation of the motor point area can be determined by surface electrical stimulation; outlining of this area is recommended as a guide to the surgeon. Intercostal muscle is an example of a muscle in which the innervation can be easily examined.

Excision of the Specimen of Muscle

It is possible in special clinics to perform muscle biopsies under local anaesthesia as an out-patient clinic procedure, but facilities for this must be excellent; otherwise, the complications of a haematoma or of sepsis are possible because of faulty surgical technique or nursing. In Oxford we have always insisted that a muscle biopsy should be carried out in the operating theatre with the normal aseptic precautions and the availability of diathermy and other common surgical resources. In this way a muscle biopsy may be quickly carried out by an experienced surgeon in optimum conditions with no likelihood of complications. The actual excision is not a simple task to be left to an inexperienced operator.

The actual size of the specimen should be $3 \times 2 \times 1$ cm in a large muscle from an adult patient. Naturally, from a small muscle or from a child, a smaller sample of muscle may have to be accepted. The rectangular block of muscle should be excised longitudinally across the motor point area. Note that the main dimension is longitudinal to the muscle and the smallest diameter is the depth of the specimen. The skin incision should be larger than the longitudinal extent of the biopsy, to enable the portion of muscle to be removed undamaged and without diathermy. It should be excised with a very sharp scalpel and with minimum handling by forceps, which can conveniently grasp the covering aponeurosis and thus avoid compressing the muscle fibres.

Consideration of the above requirements will explain why an experienced surgeon working under good conditions is essential. The skin incision must be thoughtfully planned and carefully sutured to avoid a disfiguring scar.

Initial Handling of the Specimen

The excised portion of muscle should be immediately laid on a clean white card and allowed to adhere. At this time small portions of undamaged muscle are taken into an osmium or glutaraldehyde fixation for electron microscopical preparation. A further portion is removed and plunged into liquid nitrogen to obtain a rapidly frozen block for histochemistry.

The remaining major part of the specimen is left on the card for 15 minutes, during which time the muscle fibres relax and the specimen becomes firmly stuck to the card. The card with the attached muscle is then placed in a large volume of 10 per cent neutralised formalin.

Conventional Light Microscopy

The specimen of muscle is allowed to fix, still attached to the card, in 10 per cent neutralised formalin for at least 24 hours and preferably 48 hours, after which tissue blocks for embedding are taken. The ends of the specimen are trimmed by making transverse cuts with a sharp scalpel 0.5 cm from each end; these provide suitable blocks for transverse sections. The remainder of the specimen is split longitudinally into two halves by a thick and slightly blunt scalpel, which passes between the muscle bundles rather than cutting and tearing the muscle fibres. One half provides a block for longitudinal paraffin sections and the other is used for frozen sections (see below). The L.S. and T.S. × 2 specimens are dehydrated in successive alcohol solutions, cleared with chloroform, and embedded in paraffin. Sections are cut at 7 μm and stained routinely with haematoxylin and eosin, and haematoxylin and van Gieson. A useful addition to these stains is a trichrome stain and a PAS reaction. Other stains are performed as appropriate. Celloidin embedding gives inferior results, as the sections cannot be cut as thin by the usual methods. Araldite (epoxide) embedding gives superior sections, but staining gives rise to problems which have not yet been fully overcome.

Examination of the Innervation

The most useful technique employed to demonstrate nerve axons is Schofield's modification of Bielschowsky's method. This technique is performed on serially mounted 50 μm frozen sections. (The method is given at the end of this chapter.) An alternative technique to demonstrate intramuscular nerve endings is the intravital staining of the axons in the muscle by the local injection of methylene blue prior to the muscle biopsy (Coërs and Woolf, 1959).

Histochemical Examination

A large number of histochemical techniques are available for muscle in the sense that chemical compounds or enzymes can be demonstrated in this way. For example, over 50 enzymes can be shown in muscle. However, only a few of these methods are capable of yielding useful information in the diagnosis of disease. The following routine is used on muscle biopsies in the author's laboratory in Oxford. For an extensive review the reader is referred to Pearse (1972).

At the time of the surgical excision of the portion of muscle, two small pieces, each about 1 × 0.5 × 0.5 cm, are attached to microtome chucks, one oriented for cutting longitudinally and the other transversely with respect to the muscle fibres. The method of freezing is to attach the tissue blocks directly to the microtome chuck with Ames Tissue-Tek, quench the chuck and tissue by immersion in iso-pentane, and then lower the chuck and tissue into liquid nitrogen. This procedure is much superior to the use of solid CO_2, which freezes the tissue too slowly to avoid artefacts. A supply of several litres of liquid nitrogen kept in a special insulated container will last one week. The frozen blocks can be examined immediately or kept at $-70°C$ to be examined at leisure. Cryostat sections 5 μm in thickness are cut.

The enzyme reactions for succinic dehydrogenase, for muscle phosphorylase, and for adenosine triphosphatase are carried out. The methods for these enzyme reactions are given at the end of the chapter. The periodic acid–Schiff reaction is used, and the oil-red-o dye is applied to show neutral fat.

Histochemistry can be combined with electron microscopy by the method described by Kerpel-Fronius and Hajos (1968), which demonstrates the ultrastructural location of succinic dehydrogenase activity. These methods of visualising the location of enzymes are clearly capable of further development.

Electron Microscopy

There are now several general accounts of electron microscope techniques relevant to the examination of biological tissues, and for details the reader is referred to Pease (1964) and Kay (1965). An excellent short handbook is that of Mercer and Birbeck (1966). The comments that follow are intended to help in the application of these techniques to the ultrastructural examination of human muscle biopsies.

Fixation is the first difficulty in obtaining results comparable to those seen with animal tissues in which the luxury of perfusion-fixation gives rapid controllable fixation. Human muscle, within seconds or minutes of excision, must be minced with a new razor blade on a clean plastic surface in a small pool of fixative. The aim is to obtain portions $1 \times 0.5 \times 0.5$ mm from tissue away from the surgical trauma of excision. At Oxford we have used Caulfield's solution (Caulfield, 1957) when primary osmium fixation is employed or glutaraldehyde. Both formulae are given at the end of this chapter. There is more flexibility with glutaraldehyde fixation because the increased penetrance allows a slightly larger portion of muscle to be taken. However, our own results appear to favour primary osmium fixation.

Following fixation, washing is carried out in buffer solution and dehydration in graded ethyl alcohol solutions. Embedding in Oxford is carried out in Araldite (epoxide), but elsewhere, particularly in the U.S.A., Epon and Vestopal are used. Blocks are oriented and trimmed so that the muscle fibres are cut either longitudinally or transversely. More information is usually obtained from longitudinal sections. Section cutting may be done equally well by glass or diamond knives, provided the nature of the embedded block agrees with the type of knife. Staining with uranyl acetate and lead citrate is usually carried out.

HISTOLOGICAL TECHNICAL METHODS

The modified Bielschowsky method to demonstrate axons in muscle, the histochemical methods for 3 muscle enzymes, and two fixatives for electron microscopy will be given.

Schofield's Modification of Bielschowsky's Method for Axons[*]

METHOD

1. Cut frozen sections at 50 μm.
2. Wash in 3 changes of distilled water.
3. Leave for 1–3 hours at 37° C in 50 ml of 50% alcohol to which 15 drops of pure pyridine have been added.
4. Wash in 3 changes of distilled water.
5. Leave in 20% silver nitrate in the dark at room temperature for 15–30 minutes.

[*](Smith and Beesley, 1970).

6. Blot. Transfer through:

10% neutral formalin in tap water	5 seconds
10% neutral formalin in tap water	5–10 seconds
2% neutral formalin in tap water	10 seconds

Agitate sections in each solution.

7. Rinse quickly in distilled water and blot.

8. Impregnate in 20% silver nitrate (to which ammonia has been added until the precipitate formed has just dissolved) for about 30 seconds.

9. Blot.

10. Transfer to 1% neutral formalin in tap water until the section turns brown (not black), agitating continuously.

11. Wash in distilled water for 1–2 minutes.

12. Tone, if desired, in 0.2% gold chloride.

13. Wash in distilled water.

14. Fix in 5% sodium thiosulphate for 5 minutes.

15. Wash in distilled water, mount on gelatinized slide, dehydrate, clear and mount in Xam.

Method for Succinate Dehydrogenase Activity

INCUBATING MEDIUM

0.2 M sodium succinate	5 ml
0.2 M K · H_2PO_4	1 ml
0.2 M Na_2HPO_4	4 ml
Nitro B.T. 1 mg/ml	10 ml (10 mg)
pH should be 7.2–7.6.	

METHOD

1. Mount 5 μm cryostat sections on slides.
2. Cover with approximately 0.2 ml of medium.
3. Incubate for 1 hour at 37° C.
4. Wash in distilled water.
5. Mount in glycerine jelly.

Method for Muscle Phosphorylase Activity

STOCK SOLUTION

0.1 M acetate buffer (pH 5.9)	100 ml
glucose-1-phosphate	1 g
adenosine-5-phosphate	100 mg
glycogen	20 mg

INCUBATING MEDIUM

Stock solution (filtered)	2.5 ml
ethyl alcohol	0.5 ml
insulin (40 units/ml)	1 drop

METHOD

1. Cover 5 μm cryostat sections with medium.
2. Incubate for 1 hour at 37° C.
3. Shake off surplus medium.
4. Place in Gram's iodine for 20 seconds.
5. Remove and blot.
6. Mount in iodine-glycerine 1 in 5.

Method for Adenosine Triphosphatase (ATPase)

INCUBATING MEDIUM

0.1 M sodium barbitone	2 ml
0.18 M calcium chloride	1 ml
Distilled water	7 ml

adenosine triphosphate (disodium salt) 15 mg.
When ATP is dissolved, adjust pH to 9.4 with 0.1 NaOH. Filter.

METHOD

1. Incubate sections for 30 minutes.
2. Wash for 1 minute with distilled water 3 times.
3. Place in 2% CoC_2 for 3 minutes.
4. Wash for 1 minute with distilled water 3 times.
5. Place in dilute yellow ammonium sulphide for 30 seconds.
6. Wash in distilled water.
7. Dehydrate, clear, mount in Xam.

Caulfield's O_sO_4 Fixative

BARBITONE BUFFER SOLUTION

sodium barbitone	14.7 g
sodium acetate (3 H_2O)	9.7 g
distilled water	500 ml.

Keep at 4° C.

FRESH FIXATIVE

barbitone buffer solution	5 ml
0.1 N HCl	5 ml

2% aqueous O_sO_4 20 ml
(sucrose 0.045 g for every ml)
distilled water   10 ml
Keep at 4° C. Use within 12 hours.

METHOD

1. Mince tissues into fresh, ice-cold fixative; trim if necessary.
2. Fix for 2 hours at 4° C.
3. Wash in buffer solution.
4. Dehydrate in successive alcohols and embed.

Glutaraldehyde Fixative

PHOSPHATE BUFFER SOLUTION

0.2 M Na $H_2PO_4 \cdot H_2O$.   23 ml.
    (27.6 g/1)
0.2M. $Na_2H \cdot PO_4 H_2O$ 77 ml
    (35.61 g/1)
distilled water   100 ml

FRESH FIXATIVE (4% SOLUTION)

25% aqueous glutaraldehyde w/v   4 ml
phosphate buffer solution   21 ml
Check that pH is 7.3.

METHOD

1. Mince into fresh, ice-cold 4% glutaraldehyde.
2. Allow to fix at 4° C for 4–6 hours.
3. Wash overnight in phosphate buffer solution.
4. Fix in 1% O_sO_4 in phosphate buffer for 2 hours.
5. Wash in phosphate buffer.
6. Dehydrate in alcohol.

References

Brandt, S. (1951). Werdnig-Hoffman's infantile progressive muscular atrophy. Clinical aspects, pathology, heredity and relation of Oppenheim's amyotonia congenita and other morbid conditions with laxity of joints or muscles in infants. Munksgaard, Copenhagen.

Caulfield, J. B. (1957). Effects of varying the vehicle for O_sO_4 in tissue fixation. J. Biophys. Biochem. Cytol. 3, 827–830.

Coërs, C., and Woolf, A. L. (1959). The Innervation of Muscle. Blackwell, Oxford.

Cohen, H. L., and Brumlik, J. (1968). A Manual of Electromyography. Hoeber, New York.

Ebashi, S., Toyokura, Y., Momoi, H., and Sugita, H. (1959). High creatine phosphokinase activity of sera of progressive muscular dystrophy patients. J. Biochem. (Tokyo) *46*, 103.

Hirano, A., Kurland, L. T., Krooth, R. S., and Lessell, S. (1961). Parkinsonism-dementia complex, an endemic disease on the Island of Guam. I. Clinical features. Brain *84*, 642–661.

Hirano, A., Malamud, N., and Kurland, L. T. (1961). Parkinsonism-dementia complex, an endemic disease on the Island of Guam. II. Pathological features. Brain *84*, 662–679.

Kay, D. (1965). Techniques for Electron Microscopy. 2nd ed. Blackwell, Oxford.

Kerpel-Fronius, S., and Hajos, F. (1968). The use of ferricyanide for the light and electron microscopic demonstration of succinic dehydrogenase activity. Histochemie *14*, 343–351.

Kloepfer, H. W., and Emery, A. E. H. (1969). Genetic aspects of neuromuscular disease. *In* Disorders of Voluntary Muscle. J. N. Walton (Ed.). Churchill, London.

Kugelberg, E., and Welander, L. (1956). Heredofamilial juvenile muscular atrophy simulating muscular dystrophy. Arch. Neurol. Psychiat. *75*, 500–509.

Kurland, L. T., and Mulder, D. W. (1955). Epidemiologic investigations of amyotrophic lateral sclerosis. 2. Familial aggregations indicative of dominant inheritance. Neurology. (Minneap.) *5*, 182–196; 249–268.

Lenman, J. A. R., and Ritchie, A. E. (1970). Clinical Electromyography. Pitman, London.

Licht, S. (1961). Electrodiagnosis and Electromyography. 2nd ed. Waverly Press, Baltimore.

Mercer, E. H., and Birbeck, M. S. C. (1966). Electron Microscopy, a Handbook for Biologists. 2nd ed. Blackwell, Oxford.

Norris, F. H. (1963). The E.M.G. A guide and atlas for practical electromyography. Grune and Stratton, New York.

Pearse, A. G. E. (1972). Histochemistry, Theoretical and Applied, Vol. 2. 3rd. ed. Churchill-Livingstone, Edinburgh & London.

Pease, D. C. (1964). Histological techniques for electron microscopy. 2nd ed. Academic Press, New York.

Pennington, R. J. T. (1969). Biochemical aspects of muscle disease. *In* Disorders of Voluntary Muscle. J. N. Walton (Ed.). Churchill, London.

Pratt, R. T. C. (1967). The genetics of neurological disorders. Oxford University Press, London.

Ruch, T. C., Patton, J. N., Woodbury, J. W., and Towe, A. L. (1965). Neurophysiology. 2nd ed. W. B. Saunders Company, Philadelphia.

Sibley, J. A., and Lehninger, A. L. (1949). Aldolase in the serum and tissues of tumour-bearing animals. J. Natl. Cancer Inst. *9*, 303–309.

Smith, H. M., and Beesley, R. A. (1970). Practical Neuropathology. Butterworths, London.

Van Pilsum, J. F., and Wolin, E. A. (1958). Guanidinium compounds in blood and urine of patients suffering from muscle disorders. J. Lab. Clin. Med. *51*, 219–223.

INDEX

Page numbers in *italics* refer to illustrations.